Understanding Anxiety & Depression

Simple Steps to Avoid Complications, Reduce Medical Expenses, Decrease Stress and Live a Healthy & Proactive Life

Dr. Ashley Sullivan, PharmD

Copyright © 2025 by Dr. Ashley Sullivan PharmD

All rights reserved.

No portion of this book may be reproduced in any form without written permission from the publisher or author, except as permitted by U.S. copyright law.

Contents

Introduction	1
1. The Brain Behind the Scenes: Understanding the Physiology of Anxiety and Depression	7
2. Navigating the Landscape of Anxiety and Depression Disorders	25
3. Stress Less: Overcoming the Invisible Enemy	71
4. A Closer Look at Medication: the Good, the Bad, and the Necessary	81
5. Nourishing the Mind: The Role of Nutrition in Mental Health	97
Your Voice Could Transform a Life	109
6. Journey into Mindfulness: Your Secret Weapon Against Anxiety and Depression	111
7. A Breath of Fresh Air: Exploring Aromatherapy for Anxiety and Depression	125
8. Unwind Your Mind: Exploring Relaxation Techniques for Anxiety and Depression	133
9. Nightly Nurturing: the Role of Sleep in Mental Health	151
Conclusion	157

Spreading Hope, One Review at a Time	158
References	159

Introduction

"I often wonder how many others are sitting near me, stuck in their own quiet battles with physical or mental or spiritual health, afraid or unwilling or even unable to discuss them, silently pleading for someone to extend any added amount of grace."
—— Carlee J. Hansen

I remember the first time I encountered a patient in my pharmacy who was struggling with anxiety and depression. It was a young woman, no more than twenty-five years old. She had come to my pharmacy in search of help for her mental anguish. Her hands were shaking, her eyes were full of fear, yet she managed to tell me about all the struggles she faced in her daily life due to her condition.

That moment changed me forever; it made me realize that treating anxiety and depression is more than just a bottle of pills. It's about acknowledging the depth of human experience and the profound impact that a compassionate, holistic approach can have on someone's journey toward well-being. From that point forward, I dedicated myself to understanding the nuanced layers of these conditions, exploring the role of lifestyle, nutrition, and the mind-body connection in accessing true healing. It's a journey that continues to shape my perspective, emphasizing the importance of empathy, education, and a comprehensive approach in helping individuals navigate the often challenging terrain of mental health.

It's surprising, even shocking, how widespread anxiety disorders are. In fact, an estimated 4 percent of the global population is currently struggling with anxiety. In 2019 alone, 301 million people were affected worldwide. Sadly, anxiety takes a heavy toll on individuals and communities alike. Depression isn't far behind, affecting roughly 3.8 percent of the global population. The United States sees even higher rates of depression. In 2021, 8.3 percent of adults in the U.S. were diagnosed with depression. The prevalence is higher in women than men. Tragically, for the elderly—those over sixty years of age—the numbers worldwide climb even higher, with 5.7 percent of adults over sixty dealing with depression. The gravity of these statistics can't be ignored, especially as they contribute to another troubling reality: suicide. Every year, over 700,000 people die by suicide—the fourth leading cause of death among young adults aged fifteen to twenty-nine. Clearly, improving mental health is more important than ever.

With my background as a pharmacist, integrative health coach, and functional medicine practitioner, I bring a unique and dynamic perspective to the world of healthcare. With years of professional experience under my belt, I have honed my skills in both traditional and holistic approaches, giving myself an edge in treating patients in a more comprehensive manner.

I believe that combining traditional and holistic approaches can provide a unique and comprehensive perspective when it comes to health and wellness. Traditional approaches often focus on the physical symptoms and diagnosis, while holistic approaches take a more whole-person view of the mind, body, and spirit. Together, this combination can create an approach that values both scientific rigor and the individual's experience.

When it comes to taking care of our health, it's not just about addressing physical ailments. Mental, emotional, and spiritual well-being are just as important, especially when dealing with anxiety and depression. That's where a holistic approach comes in. It's a way of looking at our health as a whole, integrating different approaches to address all aspects of ourselves.

The popularity of this perspective is growing, as more and more people realize the benefits of treating themselves as a whole person, not just a sum of parts. It's exciting to think about the possibilities that come with this approach and the many ways it can be tailored to meet each individual's unique needs.

As a pharmacist and an integrative health coach, my passion for and commitment to improving the well-being of individuals is evident in everything I do. I prioritize the empowerment of my patients in taking control of their mental health, recognizing that everyone's journey looks different. Whether it is through talk therapy, medication management, or lifestyle modifications, I strive to deliver personalized care that enables individuals to lead fulfilling lives. The work I do is incredibly rewarding, and I am constantly inspired by the resilience and strength of my patients. Together, we navigate challenging emotions and experiences, and I am proud to support them in their progress toward better mental health.

That is why this book is a labor of love and breaks the traditional mold for self-help books. This beginners' guide comprises three main parts. The first part will focus on the fundamental understanding of anxiety and depression. Here, I will delve into the causes and symptoms of these conditions, helping you to recognize and manage them effectively. In the second part, I will explore holistic approaches to help manage these conditions, including both natural and traditional Western medicine. Finally, I will focus on lifestyle factors that may contribute to anxiety and depression, such as diet, exercise, and sleep habits. I have organized the book in this clear and methodical structure to help you navigate and explore it with ease.

Struggling with mental health issues can feel debilitating, but it's important to remember that there are solutions out there that don't just involve medication. This book provides a refreshing perspective on non-pharmaceutical approaches to wellness. It's not just about theoretical ideas, but about practical advice that can be applied to your life right away. Relatable real-life examples shared throughout will help illustrate how these techniques can be incorporated into your daily routine. From meditation and yoga to spending time in nature and practicing gratitude, this book offers a wide array of practical tools and strategies to improve overall well-being. With its careful balance of theory and practice, this book is not just about information—it's about creating a safe environment where you feel secure, supported, and nurtured. Reading this book won't solve everything, but it can certainly help you gain a better understanding of your mental health so that you can make progress toward a happier, healthier life.

Let's face it, anxiety and depression can be overwhelming and confusing to navigate. That's why having a healthcare provider's perspective translated into simple, understandable words can provide a valuable sense of clarity. It's a natural instinct to want to take control of your own health and make changes that will positively impact your wellbeing. However, it's important to remember that when it comes to treating some forms of anxiety and depression, lifestyle changes may not be enough. While equally important, they should not replace the guidance of your doctor when it comes to taking prescribed maintenance medications. Failing to follow their instructions could result in recurring symptoms and even a worsening of your condition. It's crucial to maintain healthy habits, but equally important to comply with your doctor's instructions for the best possible outcome.

If you've made it this far, chances are you're interested in learning more about anxiety and depression. Maybe you're struggling with these conditions yourself, or perhaps you know someone who is. Whatever the case may be, I encourage you to join me on this journey of understanding and managing anxiety and depression. We'll encounter twists and turns, ups and downs along the way, but I truly believe that together we can make a positive difference in our lives and the lives of those around us. So why not take that first step? Let's explore, learn, and grow together as we discover effective ways to manage these conditions and take back control of our mental health.

1

THE BRAIN BEHIND THE SCENES: UNDERSTANDING THE PHYSIOLOGY OF ANXIETY AND DEPRESSION

Have you ever felt heavy worry or sadness without really understanding why? In recent decades, there's been remarkable progress in basic neuroscience, and one standout area is the research focusing on how the brain detects and responds to threats. Research in this area has found regular patterns in how the brain and behavior are connected when dealing with threats. These patterns aren't just seen in humans but also in different types of mammals.

Let's say you're walking in the woods, and suddenly, you hear a rustle in the bushes. Your brain quickly processes this as a potential threat, and you might feel a surge of fear. In this scenario, the consistent pattern researchers talk about is how the brain (detecting the rustle) and your behavior (feeling fear) are linked when facing a potential threat. This same pattern of response is observable in other mammals, like squirrels or deer, when they sense a potential danger in their environment.

Knowing these patterns extend beyond our human experience, resonating across various mammalian species, tells us that there is something going on at the most fundamental level. Therefore, to understand them, we need to deep dive into the brain itself, unraveling the brain and its role in two of the most common mental health conditions: anxiety and depression.

It's easy to overlook the fact that these conditions have roots in the physical mechanisms of our brain. But understanding the physiology behind them is key to finding the right approach to managing them. With a clear understanding of the brain's inner workings, we can develop strategies that partner with our bodies and minds to achieve better mental health. So, let's explore the brain behind the scenes and learn what it means to take control of our physiological responses to anxiety and depression.

The Brain's Blueprint: an Introduction to Its Structure and Function

The human body is a marvel of complexity, with each individual organ and system playing its own unique role in our overall health and well-being. At the heart of every human is the nervous system, a network of cells and tissues responsible for relaying messages between the brain and the body. Neural tissue is the fundamental building block of this intricate system, providing the structure and support necessary for our nerves to function as they should. Composed of specialized cells known as neurons, this tissue is responsible for everything from controlling our basic bodily functions to processing complex thoughts and feelings. Whether we are laughing with friends or learning something new, our neural tissue is constantly working behind the scenes to keep us functioning at our very best.

The brain is an incredibly complex and powerful organ that governs much of what we do without us even realizing it. It controls everything from our thoughts and emotions to our physical movements and even the workings of our internal organs. It's like a massive central computer, with the rest of our nervous system acting as a network that relays messages back and forth, allowing us to interact with the world around us. And all of this communication is made possible by the spinal cord, which carries signals down from the brain to every corner of our bodies. It's truly amazing to think about just how much our brains do for us every single day.

Similar to a supercomputer, our brain is equipped with a fast and efficient messaging system that allows us to respond to stimuli in a split-second. When you accidentally touch a hot stove, for instance, your nerves rapidly transmit a warning signal to your brain. In response, your brain quickly sends a message back to your muscles to recoil your hand away from the heat source. This process of communication between the body and brain happens so seamlessly that it's easy to take for granted the incredible coordination required for a proper response.

Have you ever thought about what goes on inside the brain of an animal that you have never seen before? As it turns out, if you understand brain anatomy, you would actually be able to deduce the likely capacities of the animal! That is because all animal brains are very similar in overall form. It's fascinating to think that the oldest structures of the brain—the parts closest to the spinal cord that develop first in utero—carry out the same functions they did for our distant ancestors.

These "old brain" functions regulate basic survival activities, such as breathing, moving, resting, and feeding, and create our experiences of emotion. Of course, mammals such as humans have more advanced brain layers that provide us with even more complex and sophisticated functions, like better memory, more sophisticated social interactions, and the ability to experience emotions.

This is where the highly developed cerebral cortex comes into play. The cerebral cortex is a truly remarkable part of the brain, responsible for everything from sensation to movement, language to decision-making. Consisting of six distinct layers of neural tissue, the cortex is divided into different regions that specialize in processing various types of information. From the visual cortex at the back of the brain that helps us see the world around us, to the prefrontal cortex at the front of the brain that is involved in planning and decision-making, each region of the cortex plays a unique role in shaping our perception of the world and guiding our behavior.

Since it plays a crucial role in how our emotions and thoughts are regulated, when it comes to managing anxiety and depression, it is essential to understand the physiological processes that determine these emotional states. Our brain health is just as important as our physical health, and learning to take care of it is the key to living a happier and healthier life.

The brain stem takes center stage as the oldest and most internal segment of the brain, responsible for overseeing fundamental life functions such as breathing, attention, and motor responses. Its journey begins at the point where the spinal cord meets the skull, giving rise to the medulla—the brain stem area governing heart rate and breathing. Interestingly, the medulla alone can sustain life in many cases; animals with the remainder of their brains disconnected above the medulla can still perform essential functions like eating, breathing, and moving. Above the medulla sits the pons, a spherical structure within the brain stem that significantly contributes to controlling body movements, particularly in terms of balance and walking.

Within the medulla and pons runs a lengthy and narrow network of neurons referred to as the reticular formation. This network acts as a gatekeeper, sifting through incoming stimuli from the spinal cord, filtering some out, and relaying the remaining signals to other regions of the brain. The reticular formation plays pivotal roles in various activities, including walking, eating, engaging in sexual activity, and sleeping. Notably, when an animal's reticular formation receives electrical stimulation, it promptly transitions to a fully awake state. Conversely, severing the reticular formation from the higher brain regions induces a deep coma in the animal.

Beyond the brain stem, there are other brain regions playing a role in shaping our behavior and emotions. One key player is the thalamus, a structure shaped like an egg located above the brain stem. The thalamus takes the baton from the brain stem and adds an extra layer of filtering to the sensory information making its way up from the spinal cord through the reticular formation. It's a gatekeeper, sorting through and refining this information. After this refining process, the thalamus passes on some of these signals to the higher levels of the brain (Sherman & Guillery, 2006).

But wait, there's more! The thalamus isn't just a middleman; it's a two-way communicator. It receives responses from the higher brain and relays them to the medulla and cerebellum, coordinating the brain's responses.

Now, when it comes to getting some shut-eye, the thalamus is your go-to guy. It takes charge by turning off incoming signals from the senses, giving us the green light to rest and recharge. In a nutshell, the thalamus is like the brain's multitasking wizard, managing information flow and ensuring our mental well-being, even while catching some Zs.

While the brain stem takes care of the basics, like motor functions and essential aspects of life, the limbic system is the maestro of memory and emotions, including our reactions to rewards and punishments. Nestled between the brain stem and the cerebral hemispheres, the limbic system is home to crucial players such as the amygdala, hypothalamus, and hippocampus.

First up, the amygdala, shaped like two almonds, pulls the strings on how we perceive and respond to aggression and fear. It's the puppet master linked to various bodily systems dealing with fear, such as the sympathetic nervous system, facial responses, smell processing, and neurotransmitter release tied to stress and aggression (Best, 2009). Studies like Klüver and Bucy's (1939), showed that tweaking the amygdala can turn an aggressive rhesus monkey into a calm one. Plus, it's the amygdala that helps us learn from fear-inducing situations, engraving the details into our brains so we steer clear in the future (Sigurdsson et al., 2007).

Moving on to the hypothalamus, which is situated just under the thalamus (hence its name). This brain structure is a multitasker, regulating hunger, sexual behavior, and connecting the nervous system with the endocrine system via the pituitary gland. It's the brain's control center for body temperature, hunger, thirst, and sex, rewarding us with feelings of pleasure when these needs are met. Olds and Milner's accidental discovery in 1954 highlighted how stimulating the hypothalamus could trigger rats to seek pleasure, even at the expense of crossing electrified grids.

Lastly, the hippocampus, with its two horn-like structures, hangs out near the amygdala. This brain region is the memory maestro, critical for storing information in long-term memory. If the hippocampus takes a hit, building new memories becomes a challenge, and the individual lives in a world where recent experiences fade away, though older memories remain untouched.

The Adaptable Brain: Exploring Neuroplasticity

Neuroplasticity refers to the brain's remarkable ability to reorganize itself and form new connections between neurons. This adaptability allows the brain to change its structure and function in response to experiences, learning, and even damage. When it comes to managing anxiety and depression, neuroplasticity becomes a powerful tool.

Training the brain involves engaging in activities or exercises that promote positive changes in neural pathways and connections. This can include practices like cognitive behavioral therapy, mindfulness, and other therapeutic interventions. These activities stimulate the brain to create new neural pathways or strengthen existing ones associated with positive thoughts and behaviors.

For example, in the context of anxiety and depression, engaging in mindfulness meditation may lead to changes in the brain's structure and function. Studies have shown that regular mindfulness practice can impact the amygdala, a region associated with emotional responses, leading to reduced reactivity to stressors. Similarly, cognitive behavioral therapy can help reframe negative thought patterns and develop healthier neural connections over time.

But how does neuroplasticity work exactly? Let's do a deep dive!

Normally, specific areas of our brains control specific areas of our lives like movement, vision, and hearing. If these areas get damaged, we might lose the ability to do those things. For example, if a baby's face-recognition area is damaged, they might struggle to recognize faces later on (Farah et al., 2000).

But here's the encouraging part—the brain isn't set in stone. Its neurons can rearrange and stretch themselves to take on new tasks or fix damage. This constant reshuffling and rewiring are what we call neuroplasticity. It's the brain's way of changing its structure and function based on experience or damage. Thanks to neuroplasticity, we can learn new things, create new memories, and adapt to new situations.

Children's brains are extremely "plastic," meaning they soak up huge amounts of information about the world. However, neuroplasticity doesn't retire in adulthood; it keeps going strong (Kolb & Fantie, 1989). This is why skilled musicians, who've fine-tuned their craft, have a larger auditory cortex and need less brain activity to play compared to beginners (Bengtsson et al., 2005; Münte, Altenmüller, & Jäncke, 2002). Our brains are a reflection of our experiences.

Now, if there's brain damage or a part of the body gets hurt, the brain steps up to the challenge. If a tumor harms the language center in the left side of the brain, the right side might pitch in to help reestablish communication (Thiel et al., 2006). If a person loses a finger, the sensory cortex adapts, and the nearby fingers become more touch-sensitive (Fox, 1984).

Here's another mind-blowing fact: while neurons can't regenerate like skin or blood vessels, recent findings show that the brain can make new neurons through a process called neurogenesis (Van Praag et al., 2004). These new neurons pop up in the deep brain and can even travel to other areas, forming new connections with other neurons (Gould, 2007).

So, even though the brain can't repair itself like magic, this research still brings hope. Scientists are now exploring ways to boost neurogenesis with drugs, aiming to rebuild damaged brains. For the purposes of mental health, neuroplasticity is very good news. It's our brain's way of saying,

"Hey, I can change and adapt!" This flexibility gives us hope for managing mental health diagnoses such as anxiety and depression in the long run. The brain is indeed a mighty, ever-changing force!

The Chemistry of Emotions: Neurotransmitters and Their Role

Have you ever felt a sudden rush of joy or a sense of calm wash over you? That could be thanks to neurotransmitters, the unsung heroes of our central nervous system. These tiny chemical messengers are constantly zipping around our brains, passing messages from one neuron to the next at lightning speed. Known as the brain's "chemical messengers," neurotransmitters play a key role in regulating our thoughts, emotions, and behaviors. From dopamine (the "pleasure" neurotransmitter) to serotonin (the "mood" neurotransmitter), they are the driving force behind some of our most powerful experiences. So the next time you're feeling a wave of happiness or an overwhelming sense of anxiety, just remember to thank your trusty neurotransmitters for their hard work.

Serotonin

Serotonin, often hailed as the "feel-good" neurotransmitter, is a key player in regulating mood, sleep, appetite, and overall well-being. Interestingly, the majority of serotonin in your body resides in the gut, specifically in the cells lining your gastrointestinal tract, accounting for about 90 percent of its presence, with only about 10 percent produced in the brain. This serotonin is released into your bloodstream where it gets absorbed by platelets.

The production of serotonin involves the essential amino acid tryptophan, which your body can't produce on its own, meaning it must be obtained through your diet. In the brain, serotonin plays a crucial role in mood regulation. Normal serotonin levels contribute to improved focus, emotional stability, happiness, and a sense of calm. Conversely, low serotonin levels are often associated with conditions such as depression, anxiety, sleep problems, digestive issues, suicidal behavior, obsessive-compulsive disorder, post-traumatic stress disorder, panic disorders, schizophrenia, and phobias.

Many medications designed to address anxiety, depression, and mood disorders focus on increasing serotonin levels in the brain.

Despite the progress in understanding serotonin, scientists still have much to discover about its role in the body and its implications for various diseases. Ongoing research aims to unravel the complexities of serotonin's functions and shed light on potential avenues for treatment and improved mental health.

Dopamine

Dopamine, often referred to as the "reward" neurotransmitter, serves as a powerful motivator, driving us to pursue goals, desires, and essential needs. When we accomplish these objectives, dopamine provides a surge of reinforcing pleasure, creating a sense of reward and satisfaction.

In instances where there is dysfunction in the dopamine system, it is associated with anhedonia, a core symptom of depression. Anhedonia is characterized by the inability to experience pleasure from activities that would typically be enjoyable. This link between dopamine dysfunction and anhedonia underscores the neurotransmitter's crucial role in our emotional well-being.

Understanding the role of dopamine sheds light on the mechanisms behind our motivation and sense of reward while highlighting its significance in mental health. Addressing dopamine-related imbalances, often through therapeutic interventions and medication, can be essential in managing symptoms of depression and restoring a sense of pleasure and fulfillment in daily life.

Norepinephrine

Norepinephrine plays a crucial role in regulating various aspects of our physiological and mental states. It is instrumental in managing stress responses, promoting alertness, and enhancing concentration. When levels of norepinephrine are out of balance, it can contribute to the development or exacerbation of anxiety disorders.

In situations where there is an overactivity or underactivity of norepinephrine, individuals may experience heightened states of arousal, restlessness, and difficulty concentrating. These imbalances are associated with symptoms commonly seen in anxiety disorders, such as excessive worry, nervousness, and a sense of being on edge.

Understanding the role of norepinephrine in the context of anxiety helps us to see the importance of maintaining a balance in neurotransmitter levels for optimal mental well-being. Addressing imbalances, often through medication or other therapeutic interventions, can be a key component in the treatment of anxiety disorders, helping individuals regain a more stable and manageable emotional state.

The Nervous System's Role: Fight-or-Flight and Its Impact

Have you ever felt your adrenaline kick in when you're faced with a stressful situation? That's because of the fight-or-flight response that's triggered by the nervous system. This response prepares your body to either fight off or run away from a potential threat. The sympathetic nervous system is responsible for activating this response, which causes an increase in heart rate, breathing rate, and blood pressure. While this response is helpful in keeping us safe in dangerous situations, chronic stress can have negative impacts on our physical and mental health. Understanding the role of the nervous system and its impact on the body can help us learn how to manage stress, and consequently our mental health, in order to maintain a healthy lifestyle.

The autonomic nervous system (ANS) is a key player in the experience of anxiety. The ANS is a division of the peripheral nervous system that controls involuntary bodily functions, including those involved in the fight-or-flight response, which is closely tied to anxiety.

The ANS has two main branches:

Sympathetic Nervous System (SNS): This branch of the ANS is responsible for activating the body's stress response. When you perceive a threat or danger, the SNS kicks in, triggering the release of stress hormones (like adrenaline and noradrenaline), increasing heart rate, dilating pupils, and preparing the body for action. This is commonly referred to as the fight-or-flight response.

Parasympathetic Nervous System (PNS): In contrast, the PNS promotes a state of relaxation and recovery. It helps bring the body back to a balanced state after the threat has passed. It's often referred to as the "rest-and-digest" response.

In situations of anxiety, the SNS can become overactive, leading to an exaggerated or prolonged stress response even in the absence of a real threat. This dysregulation of the autonomic nervous system is often associated with symptoms like increased heart rate, shallow breathing, muscle tension, and a heightened state of alertness.

Understanding the role of the autonomic nervous system in anxiety is crucial for developing strategies to manage and cope with anxious feelings.

So, as we already know, the autonomic nervous system plays a huge role in anxiety. More specifically, the fight-or-flight response is what drives our anxiety levels to dangerous heights. This primitive system was designed to keep us safe from harm, but in today's modern world, it can often work against us.

Experts say that people with anxiety disorders actually have an overactive fight-or-flight response (Purse, 2023). This means that their sympathetic nervous system is constantly on high alert, causing them to feel anxious even in completely safe situations. A study found that people with anxiety disorders had a heightened response to a stress-inducing task, compared to those without anxiety. In fact, their sympathetic nervous system was revved up to nearly double the rate of those without an anxiety disorder (Robinson et al., 2013).

But it's not just the fight-or-flight response that's at play here. The parasympathetic nervous system also plays a role in anxiety. This system helps us relax and calm down, but in people with anxiety disorders, it seems to be less active. So, what does all this mean? Essentially, it tells us that anxiety is a complex disorder that involves multiple systems in our body. It's not just a matter of "calming down" or "relaxing." In fact, some people with anxiety may not even be able to achieve a state of relaxation due to the overactivation of their sympathetic nervous system.

But there is hope. Through therapies like cognitive behavioral therapy (CBT) and Mindfulness-Based Stress Reduction (MBSR), people with anxiety can learn to better manage their symptoms and even retrain their nervous system to respond in a healthier way. It's not a quick fix, but with time and practice, it's possible to find relief from the grip of anxiety. In the upcoming chapters, we will explore the intricacies of CBT and MBSR, so stay with us.

Fight-or-flight mode can also cause physical symptoms like rapid heartbeat, sweating, or even difficulty breathing. Deep breathing and mindfulness techniques are two powerful tools that can help activate our parasympathetic nervous system, promoting relaxation and calming down our body's stress response.

Let's start with deep breathing. Simply put, deep breathing involves taking slow, deep breaths in through your nose and out through your mouth. One common technique is to inhale slowly for a count of four, hold your breath for a count of seven, and then exhale slowly for a count of eight. This breathing exercise is also known as the 4-7-8 breathing technique.

I personally like to use deep breathing when I feel overwhelmed or when I'm struggling with anxiety. For example, before giving a presentation at work, I'll take a few minutes to practice deep breathing in a quiet spot. I find it helps me slow down my racing thoughts and center myself. And it's not just anecdotal evidence—there's some scientific research that suggests deep breathing can truly help reduce anxiety. A study showed that practicing diaphragmatic breathing, a mind-body technique, can positively affect mental function (Ma et al., 2017). The findings, approached from a health psychology standpoint, have important implications for promoting mental well-being in healthy individuals.

We will take a more detailed look at the 4-7-8 breathing technique in chapter 8, including step-by-step instructions that will help you incorporate this practice into your everyday life.

Now, let's talk about mindfulness techniques. Mindfulness is all about being present in the moment and fully experiencing our thoughts and emotions—without judgment or distraction. One common mindfulness exercise is the body scan, where you focus on each part of your body, one at a time, and notice any physical sensations.

For example, let's say I'm feeling stressed at work. I might take a few minutes to sit quietly and do a quick body scan. Starting at the top of my head and moving down to my toes, I would focus on each part of my body and notice any sensations. I might notice tension in my shoulders or a knot in my stomach. By acknowledging these physical sensations, I can start to release some of the tension in my body and feel more grounded.

In a study from 2019, researchers examined the brain structure of individuals engaging in meditation for the first time. Following forty days of mindfulness meditation training, the participants experienced significant changes in their brain structures, correlating with lower depression scores. Additionally, a review by Blanck et al. (2018) concluded that practicing mindfulness on its own, without being paired with talk therapy, effectively lowers both anxiety and depression.

In chapter 6 we will look in more detail at different techniques that help to achieve the presence of mind and body encouraged through engaging in mindfulness meditation.

The Physical Manifestation: Recognizing Physiological Symptoms of Anxiety and Depression

As we mentioned in discussing fight-or-flight mode, anxiety and depression can often manifest physically too. Clenched fists, racing heartbeat, trouble sleeping, upset stomach, and sweating are just a few examples of how these conditions can impact the body. Understanding the physiological symptoms of anxiety and depression may help you recognize these conditions in yourself or others, and also seek out appropriate treatment. After all, taking care of your physical health is just as important as taking care of your mental health.

Let's take a deeper look at why these physical symptoms manifest, starting with one of the most common: rapid heart rate. This happens because when we're anxious, our bodies release adrenaline, which prepares us to respond to a perceived threat. Adrenaline can make our hearts beat faster, which some people describe as a "pounding" or "racing" feeling. Findings from a study published in the *Journal of Anxiety Disorders* confirmed that individuals with anxiety were more likely to experience cardiovascular symptoms such as rapid heart rate and palpitations. They may also experience chest pain or tightness, shortness of breath, and dizziness (Celano et al., 2016). These symptoms can be particularly frightening for individuals who don't understand that they are related to anxiety, making it feel like they're having a heart attack.

Another physical symptom of anxiety is restlessness, which can take a few different forms. Some people might feel like they can't sit still, while others might pace around or fidget. This happens because anxiety can make us feel like we need to do something to relieve the discomfort we're feeling. In some cases, people might even engage in activities like nail-biting or hair-pulling as a way of coping with restlessness.

Difficulty sleeping is another common physical symptom of anxiety and depression. This can take a few different forms as well. Some people might have trouble falling asleep, while others might wake up frequently throughout the night. Ironically, this lack of restful sleep can make anxiety worse, since we're more likely to be irritable and on-edge when we're sleep-deprived.

Finally, gastrointestinal problems are another physical symptom of anxiety and depression. This can include symptoms like stomach pains, diarrhea, and nausea. One possible explanation is anxiety can disrupt the normal functioning of the digestive system. In fact, research has shown that people with irritable bowel syndrome (IBS) are more likely to also have anxiety and depression (Savas et al., 2009).

To give you a real-life example, let's follow Clara. She detailed how she was anxious about a job interview she was preparing for. She noticed that her heart was pounding, she was having trouble sitting still and focusing, and she started to feel nauseous. Finding it difficult to concentrate on preparing, she started to question whether she should just cancel the interview altogether. We can see from Clara's physical symptoms how strongly they affected her mental health, highlighting the importance of recognizing these signs.

Likewise, when someone is struggling with depression, it can have a significant impact on their physical well-being. One common symptom of depression is weight change. For some people, depression can cause them to lose their appetite, leading to weight loss. For others, depression can cause them to turn to food for comfort, leading to weight gain.

A study published in *JAMA Psychiatry* found that people with depression and anxiety were more likely to be overweight or obese than people without these mental health conditions. The study also found that people with depression and anxiety had higher levels of inflammation in their bodies, which can lead to other health problems (Floriana et al., 2010).

Depression can also cause fatigue, making it difficult to feel motivated to exercise or even get out of bed in the morning. Insomnia or hypersomnia are also common symptoms of depression. Insomnia manifests as either experiencing difficulty falling asleep or an inability to stay asleep, leading to insufficient sleep in both cases. Hypersomnia involves excessive daytime sleepiness and prolonged nighttime sleep. Both conditions can have various causes, impacting overall well-being. This can lead to a cycle of fatigue and low energy that is difficult to break.

Physical aches and pains are prevalent in depression, with vague aches and pains frequently serving as initial indicators. These may encompass chronic joint pain, limb pain, back pain, gastrointestinal issues, fatigue, sleep disturbances, alterations in psychomotor activity, and changes in appetite. A study found that individuals with depression were more likely to report physical symptoms such as headaches, backaches, and stomach problems (Tylee et al., 2005). This suggests that physical symptoms could be an important indicator of depression and should not be overlooked as a potential sign of mental health issues. Notably, a significant proportion of individuals with depression, particularly those seeking primary care, may only present with physical symptoms, posing challenges in the diagnostic process (Trivedi, 2004).

Each of these physical symptoms can make it difficult for people to take care of themselves and maintain a healthy lifestyle. That's why it's so important for people with depression to seek treatment from a mental health professional, who can help them manage their symptoms and improve their overall health and well-being. Treatments like therapy, medication, and lifestyle changes can all be effective in treating depression and its physical symptoms.

So if you or someone you know is struggling with depression, it's important to remember there are effective treatments available. Seeking help from a mental health professional is the first step toward improving both mental and physical health.

When it comes to recognizing symptoms of anxiety and depression, it's important to first understand that these mental health conditions can present themselves in a variety of ways, and that physical symptoms are just one potential indicator of anxiety and depression. Symptoms can also be different for each individual, so recognizing them can take some observation and understanding. One way to identify these symptoms is to pay close attention to changes in behavior. For example, if a normally energetic and attentive individual starts showing signs of fatigue or a lack of interest in activities they once enjoyed, it could be a sign of depression.

2

NAVIGATING THE LANDSCAPE OF ANXIETY AND DEPRESSION DISORDERS

We saw earlier how anxiety affects the worldwide population, but did you know that more than forty million Americans over the age of eighteen suffer from an anxiety disorder? Were you aware that depression is a major contributor to mortality, morbidity, and disability in the United States (McLaughlin, 2011)? These are harrowing statistics, and this is why it's so important we understand how essential it is that we learn to recognise the symptoms and seek treatment.

If you have ever found yourself drowning in worry, fear, or sadness to the point where it takes over your thoughts and actions, you might have experienced symptoms of anxiety and depression. These disorders affect millions of people worldwide, and their prevalence has only increased in recent years. Understanding the distinct types of anxiety and depressive disorders will help you to begin navigating this complex landscape.

This chapter will explore the various symptoms, causes, and treatments, empowering readers to recognize and manage these conditions effectively. Whether you're a sufferer yourself or simply seeking to support a loved one, the insights and knowledge presented here will help you make informed decisions and seek appropriate professional help.

Unraveling Generalized Anxiety Disorder (GAD)

Have you ever found yourself stressing about every little thing, from work deadlines to whether you locked the front door? If so, you might be experiencing an anxiety disorder called generalized anxiety disorder (GAD). This condition is marked by constant worry over a multitude of different aspects of life, often leading to feelings of tension and unease. It's characterized by a constant feeling of being overwhelmed, as well as excessive, frequent, and unrealistic worries about everyday life, such as cleaning, cooking, studying, or job responsibilities. To give you an idea of what this can look like, imagine a student who spends hours every day worrying about their grades, relationships, and future job prospects, even when things seem to be going well.

GAD is a serious mental health condition that can significantly impact a person's ability to function normally. According to the Anxiety and Depression Association of America (2020), it affects approximately 6.8 million adults or 3.1 percent of the population in the United States each year, making it one of the most common mental health disorders.

Those who suffer from GAD often find that their worries and anxieties interfere with their daily lives in significant ways, making it difficult for people to carry out their normal routines. For instance, someone with GAD may struggle to get out of bed in the morning because they are consumed with worry about what might happen during the day ahead. They may have trouble concentrating at work or school because their mind is constantly racing with anxious thoughts. Some people might even find it challenging to leave their homes at all, as they worry about potential dangers or threats that could harm them or their loved ones.

Another way it can impact people's lives is by straining relationships with friends, family members, and romantic partners. Because people with this condition are constantly worried and anxious, they may become irritable or short-tempered with others, leading to arguments or conflicts. They may also seek frequent reassurance from those around them, leading to stress and frustration for their loved ones. Individuals with GAD might also have trouble trusting others or developing close relationships due to their fears and anxieties.

Studies have shown that the effects of GAD on a person's life can be quite severe (Newman, 2000). Research results confirm that people with GAD are more likely to have social and occupational impairments, such as difficulty forming and maintaining relationships, lower levels of job satisfaction, and reduced work productivity (Wittchen, 2002). There is also evidence to suggest that generalized anxiety disorder can lead to other physical and mental health problems, such as insomnia, chronic pain, and even cardiovascular disease (Martens et al., 2010).

While there is no one-size-fits-all solution to this complex mental health disorder, it is important to recognize the ways in which generalized anxiety disorder can interfere with people's lives and support those who are struggling with this condition in seeking appropriate help and treatment.

If you're dealing with GAD, you probably recognize that your anxiety is cranked up higher than the situation warrants, yet those unwarranted worries just won't let up. Physical symptoms associated with GAD can vary, but there are some common ones I come across in my practice. You might have trouble falling or staying asleep, leaving you fatigued and worn out. You might notice trembling, twitching, or tense muscles, adding to the physical toll. Headaches and irritability might become frequent companions, making it a bit tougher to get through the day. There's also excessive sweating, hot flashes, and lightheadedness, adding an extra layer of discomfort. Trouble breathing and nausea can sneak in, creating an overall sense of unease. The need for frequent urination and that persistent lump in the throat can add to the challenge.

The mental toll is significant too. Fatigue, poor concentration, and being easily startled can make it difficult to focus or relax. It's a complex mix, but it's important to remember that various strategies like cognitive behavioral therapy (CBT), medications, and complementary health approaches can help in managing these symptoms.

Treating Generalized Anxiety Disorder

CBT, or cognitive behavioral therapy, is a form of psychotherapy that supports you in recognizing and adjusting thought patterns causing anxious feelings. It taps into different methods, like tweaking thoughts through cognitive restructuring, gradually facing fears in a safe way with exposure therapy, and getting into mindfulness-based interventions to observe and accept thoughts and emotions without judgment. The goal? To cut down on anxiety and boost overall well-being.

Research has shown that CBT is an effective treatment for generalized anxiety disorders (Kaczkurkin & Foa, 2015). Participating in CBT has also shown connections to improvements in the overall quality of life for individuals managing anxiety. This therapeutic approach addresses the symptoms of anxiety and the underlying thought patterns and behaviors that contribute to the condition, creating positive changes that impact various aspects of life (Hofmann & Boettcher, 2014).

Treating GAD with CBT mainly involves working on how we think. One way is by using cognitive techniques to ease excessive worrying. In the GAD treatment manual by Craske and Barlow (2006), patients are taught to change thinking patterns that contribute to anxiety. This includes questioning thoughts that make risks seem bigger than they really are and figuring out how to shift anxious thinking to more helpful thoughts. For example, a person with GAD may have a tendency to catastrophize, or imagine worst-case scenarios, in situations that are not actually dangerous. Through cognitive restructuring, a person can learn to challenge these catastrophic thoughts and replace them with more realistic and helpful statements. This can reduce anxiety and increase feelings of control and confidence.

When it comes to CBT for GAD, several techniques are employed to target maladaptive thought patterns and behaviors:

Cognitive Restructuring

Many people go through occasional bouts of negative thought patterns, but when these patterns dig in too deep, they can interfere with relationships, accomplishments, and overall well-being. That's where cognitive restructuring steps in. These are a set of therapeutic techniques designed to help people recognize and shift those negative thinking patterns.

Sometimes, I too find myself caught up in cognitive distortions—those funky thought patterns that skew how I see things. They often bring on feelings of depression, anxiety, mess with my relationships, and sometimes lead me down a self-defeating path. Some examples of these thought patterns include black-and-white thinking, catastrophizing, overgeneralization, and personalization. That's where cognitive restructuring comes in for me. It's a chance to catch those not-so-great thoughts as they pop up and work on reframing them into something more accurate and helpful. The idea is, if I can shift how I see certain events or situations, it might just change up the feelings and actions that follow. By examining the evidence for and against these thoughts, I can develop more balanced and realistic perspectives, thereby reducing emotional distress and improving well-being (Gakinya, Wasanga, & Kipnusu, 2022).

Cognitive restructuring and problem-solving have been used as prevalent strategies in CBT programs targeting depressive symptoms, highlighting their significance in therapeutic interventions (Fréchette-Simard, Plante, & Bluteau, 2018). Cognitive restructuring has also shown long-term effectiveness in preventing relapse after short-term treatment for major depressive disorder, suggesting its pivotal role in sustained recovery (Hensley, Nadiga, & Uhlenhuth, 2004). Similarly, in treating anxiety disorders in children and adolescents, cognitive restructuring, alongside other CBT strategies, demonstrated a significant effect in remission rates compared to control groups (Cartwright-Hatton, et al. 2004).

So, in a nutshell, cognitive restructuring is like having a mental toolkit for turning those "I can't do anything right" thoughts into an "I can totally handle this" attitude. It's backed by science and has helped many people feel better and more in control of their feelings.

So, how do you actually restructure a negative thought?

Self-Monitoring

In order to break free from an unproductive thought pattern, it's crucial to pinpoint the mistake you're making. Cognitive restructuring relies on your ability to detect those thoughts that trigger negative feelings and states of mind.

It's also beneficial to pay attention to when and where these thoughts arise. You might find that you're more susceptible to cognitive distortions in specific situations. Identifying those circumstances can give you a heads-up and help you prepare in advance.

Suppose you're someone who often experiences social anxiety. You might notice a recurring cognitive distortion when attending social events. Your thought pattern could be something like, "Everyone at the party will find me awkward and boring. No one will want to talk to me, and I'll end up feeling like an outsider."

When you recognize this tendency, it will allow you to be proactive in challenging and changing that negative thought before entering social situations. It's about understanding your vulnerability and using self-monitoring to shift your thought patterns toward more positive and realistic perspectives.

Challenging Your Assumptions

Keep the previous example of experiencing social anxiety in your mind. We will take that along as we go through the steps involved in cognitive restructuring.

Challenging your assumptions is a crucial part of cognitive restructuring, as it helps you overcome thoughts that hinder a productive life. A therapist using cognitive restructuring techniques might introduce Socratic questioning to help you identify biases or illogical aspects in your automatic thoughts.

Here are some questions they might ask you to consider:

- Is this thought based on emotion or facts?

- What evidence supports this thought's accuracy?

- What evidence contradicts this thought's accuracy?

- How can I test this belief?

- What's the worst-case scenario, and how can I respond to it?

- What other interpretations exist for this information?

- Is this situation really black-and-white, or are there shades of gray?

Going back to the example we discussed in self-monitoring, imagine you're someone who often feels anxious before attending social events, plagued by the thought we discussed there: "Everyone at the party will find me awkward and boring. No one will want to talk to me, and I'll end up feeling like an outsider." This kind of unproductive thought pattern is a prime example of cognitive distortions—specifically catastrophizing, where you anticipate the worst possible outcome, and mind reading, where you assume you know what others are thinking. To combat this, it's crucial to first recognize when and where these thoughts typically arise, which in this case would be shortly before social gatherings.

The next step involves preparing yourself to challenge these distortions. Begin by reminding yourself that people attend social events for various reasons, including their own desire to connect and enjoy, and not everyone will be focused on judging you. Reflect on past events where you had meaningful interactions or received compliments, which serves as evidence against your distorted thoughts. Develop a more balanced thought, such as, "While I might feel awkward at times, there are people who find my company enjoyable. Not everyone will connect with me, and that's okay. It's an opportunity to meet those who do."

Generating a Fresh Perspective

Generating a fresh perspective, especially when stuck in a rut of negative thinking or facing a seemingly insurmountable challenge, involves stepping out of your current mental framework and looking at the situation anew. This can be particularly helpful in personal growth, problem-solving, and creative endeavors.

Often, the biggest hurdle to overcoming a problem or enhancing personal development is our own perspective. We get trapped in a single way of thinking, limiting our potential solutions and growth opportunities. Recognizing the need for a fresh perspective is the first step toward meaningful change. It's about acknowledging that the current way of viewing things might not be the only or the best way.

Here's how you can approach this process:
1. **Seek diverse inputs and change your environment.** For example, surrounding yourself with people who have different backgrounds, experiences, and viewpoints and engaging in discussions with them can introduce you to new ways of thinking and challenge your existing beliefs. Sometimes, a physical change can stimulate mental change. This could be as simple as rearranging your workspace, taking a different route on your walk, or traveling to a

new place. New environments can spark new ideas and insights.

2. **Adopt a beginner's mindset.** Approach problems or situations as if you know nothing about them, no matter your level of expertise. This mindset encourages curiosity and openness, leading to innovative solutions.

3. **Reflect through journaling.** Writing about your experiences and thoughts can help you see them from a different angle. It's a process of self-reflection that can reveal hidden assumptions and biases in your thinking.

4. **Practice mindfulness and meditation.** We've discussed the power of mindfulness already, and we will be discussing this in greater detail in chapter 6. These practices help in clearing your mind, reducing stress, and improving focus. A calm and focused mind is more adept at thinking creatively and viewing problems in a new light.

5. **Engage in creative activities.** Creativity isn't just for artists. Engaging in any creative activity, like painting, writing, or playing music, can help break conventional thinking patterns and inspire a fresh outlook.

Implementing the New Perspective

Once you've gained a new perspective, the challenge is to integrate it into your thinking and decision-making processes. This involves being open to changing your previous plans or beliefs based on the new insights gained. It's important to maintain flexibility in your thought process and be willing to experiment with new ideas. Adopting a new perspective can have a profound impact on your life. It can enhance problem-solving skills, boost creativity, improve relationships, and increase personal satisfaction. By seeing the world through a fresh lens, you can uncover opportunities and solutions that were previously hidden. This journey toward a new viewpoint is an ongoing process of learning, unlearning, and relearning.

Generating a fresh perspective is not just about finding a new way to look at things; it's about creating a more open, curious, and flexible mindset that welcomes change and embraces the complexity of the world. With this approach you can navigate life's challenges more effectively and enjoy a richer, more fulfilling experience.

In the wise words of Dr. Lucas D. Shallua, "Paradigm shift is for the mindful; but those who refuse to adopt to new ways of looking at things will always catch yesterday's train, flight, or bus" (Shallua 2024).

Mindfulness Techniques for Generalized Anxiety

Stress is a universal experience in our daily lives, impacting everyone regardless of age, size, or our approach to thinking and doing, whether we're contemplative or hands-on. Even those well-versed in meditation or individuals emanating tranquility through yoga encounter this unavoidable aspect of being human. As Jane Wagner puts it, "Reality is the leading cause of stress amongst those in touch with it" (Wagner 1985).

But what happens when there's too much stress? Everywhere and all at once?

Acceptance and Commitment Therapy

This is where mindfulness therapy offers a game-changing perspective; a perspective of acceptance and compassion. Forsyth and Eifert (2016) champion the powerful idea of breaking free from our endless battle with anxiety, not through force or avoidance, but through openness and acceptance. Imagine a world where anxiety is recognized as a natural part of our emotional range, no longer an enemy to conquer but a presence to meet without resistance. This therapeutic journey is not about impulsive reactions to our inner waves, but a deliberate path that nurtures self-compassion—a gentle understanding that teaches us to embrace ourselves, even in challenging times. As we embrace this mindful approach, we pave the way toward a life not ruled by anxious ups and downs, but characterized by emotional resilience.

Imagine you're standing at the edge of a diving board, the high one. Your heart's racing, palms sweating, and the water below feels like a world away. That's how living with anxiety can feel. But what if, instead of stepping back, you take a deep breath and dive in? That's the core of acceptance and commitment therapy (ACT). It's about seeing that racing heart not as an enemy, but as a part of your journey. You acknowledge the fear, but then you focus on what really matters to you, like making friends or sharing your ideas, and you take the plunge into activities that align with those values. With ACT, as Forsyth & Eifert (2016) suggest, you're not trying to outswim the shark of anxiety; instead, you're learning to swim with it. Each little victory is a step toward a richer life, with anxiety becoming just another sound in the room, not the one that drowns out all the rest.

In the dance with anxiety, ACT shows us a graceful three-step routine: accept, choose, and take action. Picture yourself stuck in a quicksand of worry, every struggle sinking you deeper. It's exhausting, right? That's where the sweet relief of mindfulness comes into play. It teaches us to acknowledge our nerves without adding fuel to the fire.

Take Jamie, for instance; public speaking used to be his kryptonite. By embracing mindfulness through ACT, Jamie learned not just to live with that knot in the stomach, but to gently nod at it and move on. He shifted the focus to personal values, such as craving deeper connections, which sparked the courage to leap into new experiences, like joining a toastmasters club, a place where stutters and shakes were met with nods and applause. For Jamie, it was not about wrestling anxiety down; it was about changing how he interacted with it.

The real power move in ACT is taking small but mighty steps toward actions that echo our values, even when anxiety tags along. This strategy doesn't mute the anxiety; instead, it amplifies our life's volume until those pesky worries fade into the background hum. It's an educated, compassionate embrace of our inner tumult enabling us to live more fully, one mindful step at a time.

The Three Senses

Have you ever found yourself swept away by the torrents of thought, so engrossed in the whirlwind of daily life that the present moment seems like a blurry footnote? The art of mindfulness can elevate our awareness to the vivid details of our immediate experiences, carving out an oasis of tranquility in the arid deserts of our bustling routines. Here's a gentle nudge toward cultivating presence: consider the sensory triad of sound, sight, and touch. Slow down, take a deep, calming breath, and ask yourself, with genuine curiosity:

- What are three things I can hear? It could be the subtle ticking of a wall clock, the distant hum of traffic filtering through the window, or the soft rhythm of your own breathing.

- What are three things I can see? Observe the intricate patterns on the nearest surface, the play of light as it dances across the room, or the simple beauty of pedestrians going by your window.

- What are three things I can feel? Notice the steadfast support of the chair beneath you, the stability of the ground anchoring your feet, or the familiar texture of a cherished object in your pocket.

I recall, on one particularly frazzled afternoon at my favorite café, the profound peace that settled over me as I engaged in this practice. Occasional stresses melted away, replaced by the harmony of jazz resonating softly, the visual serenade of an environment rich with color and life, and the tactile reassurance of my immediate surroundings. This understated yet powerful exercise rooted me back to the present, equipped with the serenity needed to face the remainder of the day's challenges.

Inviting yourself to truly experience these sensations one by one can act like an anchor, hauling your drifting attention back to the shores of the now. It's a compassionate gift to yourself, a slice of tranquility served amidst life's symphony, allowing you to reconnect with the beautiful world around you, and within.

Did you notice how I slightly changed my writing style here to include descriptive words that incorporated my senses? Using descriptive words can have a profound impact on our connection with our senses, so when you journal, use words that vividly describe what you're experiencing, even if it's all in your imagination.

It is important to recognize that these CBT techniques are not standardized; rather, they are adapted to the uniqueness of the individual's needs and experiences. Various studies, including those provided by Newman et al. (2019), consistently emphasize this characteristic of CBT, which reveals its flexibility and personalization to address the symptoms of GAD. Therefore, the combination of cognitive restructuring, mindfulness, exposure therapy, behavioral activation, and structured worry time presents therapeutic options to individuals with GAD. These techniques focus on tackling the multiple factors contributing to anxiety and address evidence-based strategies in a structured and collaborative way.

We know that GAD, if left untreated, can severely damage a person's mental and physical well-being. Fortunately, medications such as antidepressants, benzodiazepines, and beta-blockers can help manage the physical symptoms of GAD. These medications function by inducing alterations to some brain chemicals and neurotransmitters' functions, which can alleviate anxiety and fear. While no medication will completely cure GAD, they are still an effective approach to managing symptoms and improving patients' quality of life. We will look at the different options in more detail in chapter 4.

Moreover, it is important to mention that it is a good idea to consult a healthcare professional to craft personalized plans. Please do not ever take medication for anxiety or any mental health condition unsupervised. It is also vital to mention that while traditional therapy and medications can be beneficial, complementary therapies such as deep breathing, yoga, and progressive muscle relaxation can also be extremely useful.

Demystifying Major Depressive Disorder (MDD)

Have you ever had a persistent feeling of sadness that lasts for months? Or maybe you've lost interest in activities that you once enjoyed? If so, you may be one of the 8.3 percent of U.S. adults who have experienced at least one major depressive episode. Also known as clinical depression, major depressive disorder (MDD) is a severe mood disorder that can impact every aspect of daily life. It's not just a case of feeling sad or going through a tough time, but a genuine illness that affects thinking, behavior, and physical health. Luckily, there are treatment options available for MDD, and demystifying the condition is the first step toward healing.

It's crucial to emphasize the diverse and often complex nature of major depressive disorder symptoms. Let's dive into a more detailed understanding.

If you've been feeling really down, you're not alone. Depression is a bit like a shadow that colors everything in shades of gray, making even your favorite activities seem dull. It's more than just a bad day; it's feeling stuck in a sad, anxious, or empty mood that just doesn't lift.

You might notice you're not really into things you used to love, whether that's hanging out with friends, diving into hobbies, or even something like enjoying a good meal. Speaking of meals, you might find your appetite flip-flops. Some people find they're not hungry at all, while others might eat a lot more than usual. And sleep? That's all over the place too. Maybe you're tossing and turning all night or, on the flip side, sleeping way more than you need but still feeling tired.

Maybe you also feel like you're moving through molasses, with everything just slowing down? Or maybe you're on the other end, feeling super restless or irritable, like you can't sit still. That's depression interfering with your energy levels, making you feel exhausted or wound up almost all the time.

Then there's that really tough side to it—the all-encompassing feeling of worthlessness, or carrying around a lot of guilt over things that aren't even your fault. And making decisions? Even the small ones feel like climbing a mountain. Your brain is foggy and you can't think straight.

The scariest part can be thoughts about death or suicide. That's when you know it's time to get help right away. These thoughts are serious and you don't have to deal with them alone.

If you're nodding along to five or more of the aspects of MDD I've just mentioned, and they've been your constant companions for a couple of weeks, then chances are you might be dealing with depressive symptoms. Please note that the information in this book is not intended to diagnose a certain mental health condition. Use it only as a guide and consult a mental health professional if you think you might have MDD.

Having MDD doesn't mean you're weak or flawed in character. It's not about personality but about what's happening in your brain and body. Depression's got its roots in a mix of brain chemistry, genes, and what life throws at you. It's a real medical condition, which means it needs understanding, care, and the right kind of help.

The treatment approach for major depressive disorder often involves a comprehensive strategy that encompasses various modalities that address both the physiological and psychological aspects of the condition. Let's look at these in more detail.

Antidepressants

Antidepressants are a group of medications designed to help smooth out the rough edges of depression. Imagine your brain as a bustling city where messages are constantly being sent back and forth. Sometimes, in the world of depression, this messaging system gets a bit disordered. Antidepressants step in to help adjust the flow of these messages, specifically targeting neurotransmitters, those chemical messengers in the brain that we explained in chapter 1.

There are a few different types that focus on different aspects of the brain's chemistry. SSRIs, or selective serotonin reuptake inhibitors, are like the city's traffic controllers for serotonin, making sure it sticks around longer to keep a person's mood more stable. SNRIs, or serotonin and norepinephrine reuptake inhibitors, do a similar job but for two neurotransmitters: serotonin and norepinephrine. Then there are others like tricyclic antidepressants and monoamine oxidase inhibitors (MAOIs) that work in their unique ways to help lift the fog of depression.

Taking antidepressants isn't like flipping a light switch; it's more like gradually turning up the dimmer on a light. It can take some time for them to kick in, and finding the right one can be a bit of a journey. But for many, they can be a key part of the toolbox for managing depression, helping to bring back a sense of balance and hope.

Take Emma, for instance, a thirty-five-year-old graphic designer who has been struggling with depression for several months. She used to enjoy painting, hiking with friends, and attending local art classes. However, since her depression worsened, she finds it hard to motivate herself to participate in these activities. She often feels too tired after work and prefers to spend weekends alone at home, which only seems to deepen her sense of isolation and sadness. Recognizing that she needs help to break this cycle, she decides it's time for change. She talks with her doctor and ends up getting prescribed an SSRI. Over time, Emma starts to notice a lift in her mood and a decrease in those heavy feelings of sadness. This can help manage her symptoms and improve her quality of life.

Psychotherapy and Behavioral Activation

Psychotherapy for depression is like having a skilled navigator helping you steer through stormy emotional seas. It's a safe space where you can talk about anything that's weighing you down, explore your thoughts and feelings, and start to see things in a new light.

There are a few different types of therapy that are particularly good for tackling depression. Let's start with behavioral activation (BA). BA is a therapeutic approach designed to combat depression by encouraging individuals to engage in activities they find meaningful or enjoyable. The basic premise is that by increasing engagement in positive activities, individuals can improve their mood and reduce depressive symptoms.

At its core, BA encourages individuals to gradually engage in activities that are aligned with their values and interests, even when they don't initially feel like it. For example, taking up or resuming a hobby such as gardening, reading, gaming, painting, or writing. The underlying theory suggests that depression often involves a vicious cycle of inactivity and avoidance, which BA aims to break. By engaging in rewarding activities, individuals can disrupt this cycle, leading to improvements in mood and reductions in depressive symptoms.

Research supports BA's effectiveness across diverse settings and populations. A review by Soucy and Provencher (2013) highlighted BA's potential as a low-intensity, guided self-help treatment for mild to moderate depression. This finding is crucial because it suggests that BA can be disseminated widely, offering a practical and accessible option for those facing barriers to traditional therapy.

Further, BA has shown promise in treating children and adolescents with depression and anxiety (Martin & Oliver, 2018). This adaptability to younger populations underscores BA's foundational appeal: activities can be tailored to fit individual interests and developmental stages, making it a versatile approach for various ages.

It's interesting to note that emerging research suggests BA can also promote health behaviors too, such as substance use reduction and improved medication adherence, in individuals with depression (May, Litvin, & Allegrante, 2022). This expansion of BA's application areas offers promising avenues for integrating mental health and physical health interventions. Let's take another look at Emma's story. Along with taking medication, Emma's doctor recommends that she sees a therapist, who introduces her to behavioural action. Let's look at the steps she took from her initial assessment to long-term strategies:

Step 1: initial assessment with a therapist. Emma has her first visit with a therapist. Together, they identify activities that used to bring her joy and satisfaction but have been neglected due to her depression.

Step 2: activity monitoring. Emma is asked to keep a daily log of her activities and rate each activity on a scale from one to ten in terms of the pleasure she derives from it and the sense of achievement it provides. This helps both Emma and her therapist understand her current activity patterns and their impact on her mood.

Step 3: setting goals. Based on Emma's activity log, the therapist helps her set small, achievable goals for engaging in more activities. They start with low-effort activities that Emma feels she can manage, such as sketching for fifteen minutes after dinner or taking a short walk around the block twice a week.

Step 4: gradually increasing activity levels. As Emma starts to engage in these activities, she and her therapist review her activity log and how these actions affect her mood. Encouraged by small successes, Emma agrees to reintroduce more demanding activities into her routine, such as completing a small painting project or attending a weekend art class.

Step 5: tackling avoidance and planning for obstacles. Emma and her therapist work together to identify patterns of avoidance and develop strategies to overcome these barriers. For example, when Emma feels too anxious to attend an art class alone, they arrange for a friend to join her for the first few sessions.

Step 6: maintaining and expanding gains. Over time, as Emma becomes more active and begins to see improvements in her mood, she and her therapist develop a long-term plan to maintain these gains. They introduce new activities into her schedule, such as volunteering at a local community center, to continue building her sense of achievement and connectedness.

After several weeks of behavioral activation therapy, Emma notices a significant improvement in her mood. She feels more energetic, experiences a renewed interest in her hobbies, and reports feeling less isolated. While she still has challenging days, Emma now has the tools and strategies to manage her depression more effectively. This example illustrates how behavioral activation helps individuals break the cycle of depression through engagement in meaningful activities, thereby improving their mood and overall well-being.

Psychotherapy and Cognitive Behavioural Therapy

Just as we saw in dealing with generalized anxiety disorder, cognitive behavioral therapy (CBT) is an effective treatment for MDD. It works like a detective for your thoughts, helping you identify and challenge the negative thought patterns that keep you stuck in a rut, and replacing them with more balanced ones. It's all about changing how you think to change how you feel.

How Can Cognitive Behavioral Therapy Improve Depressive Symptoms?

Cognitive behavioral therapy can be used in depression much like it can in anxiety. With its structured, time-limited approach that dives into the interplay between thoughts, feelings, and behaviors, tweaking how you perceive and react to life's curveballs, CBT can help to lift the heavy fog of depressive symptoms.

This therapeutic technique isn't just for adults. Studies show it's a game-changer for children and adolescents wrestling with anxiety and depressive disorders. Whether it's one-on-one or in a group, CBT has been seen to significantly dial down gloominess, showing medium to large effects in symptom reduction (Compton, March, Brent, Albano, Weersing, & Curry, 2004). Research diving into the long-term use of CBT for depression has found that it doesn't just help you bounce back; it arms you with the tools to keep the blues at bay in the long haul (Hensley, Nadiga, & Uhlenhuth, 2004).

And guess what? CBT's adaptability doesn't end in the therapist's office. Digital platforms delivering CBT have opened new doors for treating depression, offering a promising alternative for those who might find traditional therapy settings a hurdle (Kaltenthaler, Parry, Beverley, & Ferriter, 2008).

One effective CBT technique for tackling depression is the "thought record." This technique helps individuals identify, challenge, and change negative or unhelpful thoughts, which are often a significant part of depression. Here's how it works:

Step 1: trigger identification. First, you identify a situation or moment that brought on negative feelings. This could be an event, a specific interaction, or even a memory. Let's say, for example, that Alex, a forty-five-year-old banking executive, felt a surge of sadness after a meeting at work where he felt his ideas were ignored.

Step 2: capture initial thoughts. Next, Alex writes down the automatic thoughts that popped into his head during that situation. These might be things like, "I'm not good at my job" or "Nobody respects my contributions."

Step 3: identify emotions and rate intensity. Alex then names the emotions he felt during the situation, such as sadness, frustration, or worthlessness, and rates their intensity on a scale from 0 to 100.

Step 4: analyze the evidence. This step involves examining the evidence that supports Alex's initial thoughts and the evidence against those thoughts. For example, he might recognize that his colleagues have praised his work in the past, indicating that his thoughts might not be entirely accurate.

Step 5: develop balanced thoughts. After weighing the evidence, Alex works on creating a more balanced or rational thought. Instead of thinking, "I'm not good at my job," a more balanced thought might be, "Even though my ideas weren't acknowledged in this meeting, I've received positive feedback before. It's possible my colleagues were focused on other aspects today."

Step 6: re-rate emotion intensity. Finally, Alex re-rates the intensity of his emotions after considering the more balanced thoughts. Often, individuals find that their emotional distress decreases when they view the situation in a more balanced way.

By repeatedly using the thought record technique, individuals learn to challenge and change their negative thought patterns, leading to improvements in mood and reductions in depressive symptoms. It's a practical tool that empowers people to become more aware of their thought processes and to actively reshape their thinking toward a more positive outlook.

Other Psychotherapy Options

There are other therapies available, such as interpersonal psychotherapy (IPT), which zooms in on your relationships and social interactions. It's built on the idea that improving how we communicate and relate to others can significantly lift our mood.

Then there is psychodynamic therapy, which is a bit like going on an archaeological dig into your past. It aims to uncover the root causes of your depression, helping you understand the unresolved issues or conflicts from your past that might be influencing your current feelings.

However, no matter which type of therapy you go for, the goal is to give you the tools and insights to navigate your way out of depression. It's about building resilience, finding new ways to cope with life's ups and downs, and ultimately, helping you reclaim a sense of joy and purpose.

Lifestyle Changes

Lifestyle changes can be a powerful tool in improving depressive symptoms, offering a complement to therapy and medication. Let's dive into how regular physical activity and a healthy diet can make a difference:

Regular Physical Activity

How It Helps: Lace up those sneakers because getting moving is more than just good for your body; it's great for your mood too. Exercise kicks off a release of endorphins—those feel-good chemicals that can lift your spirits. It also helps dial down the stress hormones that can weigh heavily on your mind. Plus, tiring yourself out a bit during the day can help you get better sleep at night.

Example: Alex decided during therapy sessions that he could help fight the funk by fitting regular walks into his daily schedule. Whether it's a stroll through the neighborhood or a nature hike, these walks aren't just good for his heart—they're a natural mood booster, helping him feel more grounded and less tangled up in negative thoughts.

Healthy Diet

How It Helps: What's on your plate can play a role in how you feel. Foods packed with omega-3 fatty acids, antioxidants, and essential vitamins don't just nourish your body; they support brain health too. Omega-3s, for example, are like brain food that can help combat the blues, while antioxidants fight off stress-inducing oxidative damage.

Example: As Emma worked on expanding her gains in behavioral action therapy, she took a close look at her eating habits and decided to make some changes. She started loading up on leafy greens, colorful fruits, and fish rich in omega-3s. She noticed that as she fed her brain the nutrients it needs to support a more stable mood, her sense of well-being increased.

Incorporating these lifestyle changes, along with others such as regular sleep and investing time in a hobby, doesn't mean overnight miracles, but over time, they can significantly contribute to alleviating depressive symptoms. Like any good habit, the key is consistency. So, whether it's choosing a salad over fast food or opting for a bike ride instead of a TV binge, these choices can add up to a brighter outlook on life. The role of gut health and its link to your mental health cannot be overstated. To learn more about the powerful role your gut plays in your mental health, check out my book *Understanding Leaky Gut and Digestive Health*, available on Amazon.

Supportive Therapies

Supportive therapies, particularly mindfulness-based interventions, have emerged as a valuable complement to traditional treatments for depressive symptoms, blending seamlessly with medical and psychological approaches to encourage holistic well-being.

Mindfulness practices, such as those mentioned at the end of chapter 1, offer a unique way to dial down the noise of daily stressors by promoting a state of relaxation and present-moment awareness. These practices encourage us to observe our thoughts and feelings without judgment, akin to watching clouds drift across the sky. This approach to mental health cultivates a grounding and calming effect, which can be especially beneficial for those navigating the turbulent waters of depression.

For instance, consider Lina who has been diagnosed with generalized anxiety disorder. Through conversations with her therapist, she decides to weave daily mindfulness meditation into the fabric of her life. Each morning, she carves out a quiet sanctuary where she can sit undisturbed, close her eyes, and focus intently on her breathing. This ritual is far from a mere pause in her day; it's a foundational practice that equips her with resilience and a more profound capacity to manage stress. By dedicating a few minutes to mindfulness each day, Lina has noticed a shift in her overall mood and ability to cope with life's challenges, underscoring the powerful role that supportive therapies can play in the journey toward mental health recovery.

Collaborative Care

Collaborative care represents a gold standard approach to treating MDD, recognizing that the condition's complexity often requires a variety of treatments working together with a team of healthcare professionals. At the heart of this multidisciplinary approach is the collaboration among psychiatrists, psychologists, primary care providers, and other specialists. This teamwork ensures that every angle of an individual's condition is considered, creating a holistic and personalized treatment plan.

Take Emma, for example. Her journey through depression isn't navigated with a one-size-fits-all map. Instead, her care team—a dedicated assembly of mental health professionals and medical practitioners—comes together to craft a route that's tailored just for her. They integrate medication to balance the brain's chemistry, psychotherapy to navigate the mental and emotional aspects, and lifestyle changes to support overall well-being.

This multifaceted strategy acknowledges that the roots of depression are diverse, and so too must be the methods to address it. By customizing the treatment to Emma's specific circumstances and regularly fine-tuning the approach based on her progress and feedback, the collaborative care model enhances the effectiveness of the treatment and empowers her on her path to recovery.

As a health coach, this is precisely the type of approach I take in my work. Whole-person care is at the heart of my philosophy to blend science, compassion, and individualized strategies to support each client's unique healing journey. Whether addressing physical, mental, or emotional health, I believe that the most impactful outcomes arise from integrating diverse expertise and perspectives. This alignment with the collaborative care model reflects my commitment to holistic and personalized care, ensuring that no aspect of an individual's well-being is overlooked. It's a testament to the power of collective expertise, compassion, and coordinated care in transforming the landscape of mental health treatment.

Exploring Panic Disorder: More than Just Panic Attacks

Panic disorder is not just about experiencing panic attacks. It's a complex mental health condition that can severely impact an individual's quality of life. According to the Anxiety and Depression Association of America, six million adults in the U.S. experience panic disorder, which accounts for 2.7 percent of the population. This disorder is not simply feeling anxious or sensitive; it's a real and debilitating condition that can cause intense fear, palpitations, sweating, shaking, and shortness of breath. It's important for those who experience panic disorder to understand they are not alone and that help is available. Seeking professional support can make a world of difference in managing this condition and improving overall mental health.

Panic attacks can be incredibly intense and overwhelming experiences. The sudden onset of physical symptoms, such as rapid heartbeat, sweating, and trembling, can leave you feeling trapped and helpless. Unfortunately, for some people, the fear of having another panic attack can become so consuming that they start to avoid situations or places they associate with previous attacks. This avoidance behavior can escalate quickly and start to limit one's life. For instance, someone who develops agoraphobia may end up unable to leave their house or be in public spaces without experiencing debilitating anxiety. This can lead to feelings of isolation and depression that can be hard to shake.

If you or someone you know is struggling with panic attacks or avoidance behavior, it's important to seek help from a mental health professional to learn coping strategies and techniques that can help manage symptoms and lead to a better quality of life.

Panic disorder, while a challenging condition to cope with, can be well-managed through a combination of different treatment options. Psychotherapy sessions can help to understand the root cause of panic attacks and develop coping mechanisms to manage them. Medication, such as selective serotonin reuptake inhibitors (SSRIs) and benzodiazepines, can also be prescribed by a healthcare professional to help reduce the frequency or intensity of panic attacks. Additionally, self-care practices, such as mindfulness meditation and regular exercise, can promote overall wellbeing and help to develop a greater sense of control over mental health. While it may take some time to determine which combination of treatments works best for each person, know that there is hope for you or someone you know who is living with this disorder.

Let's delve into a more detailed exploration of how psychotherapy, specifically cognitive behavioral therapy (CBT), medications, and lifestyle adjustments can play pivotal roles in managing panic attacks.

How Can Cognitive Behavioral Therapy (CBT) Improve Symptoms of Panic Disorder?

As we saw earlier, cognitive behavioral therapy focuses on the intertwined nature of thoughts, feelings, and behaviors, and how altering one can significantly impact the others. This approach is particularly beneficial in tackling panic attacks, as it delves deep into the roots of panic, offering a structured path to understanding and overcoming the intense fear and discomfort panic attacks bring and providing practical tools for change.

One of the first steps in CBT is helping individuals pinpoint the triggers of their panic attacks. These triggers can be wide-ranging, from specific thoughts that spiral into fear, situations that evoke a sense of danger, or even physical sensations that mimic the onset of an attack. By identifying these triggers, individuals can begin to understand the patterns of their panic attacks, setting the stage for intervention.

As we discussed earlier, central to CBT is the process of restructuring negative thoughts. Panic attacks are often fueled by irrational beliefs and catastrophic thinking, where the mind jumps to the worst possible conclusions. CBT challenges these thought patterns, encouraging individuals to question the reality of their fears and the likelihood of their worst fears coming true. By replacing these distorted thoughts with more realistic and balanced ones, the grip of panic begins to loosen and individuals find new ways to engage with their thoughts that don't escalate into panic.

Take John, for instance, who often experiences panic attacks in situations where he feels trapped, such as during meetings at work or in crowded elevators. His panic is driven by the thought, "If I have a panic attack here, it will be disastrous. I'll be utterly humiliated, and everyone will judge me." This thought spirals into intense fear, increasing his risk of experiencing a panic attack.

In CBT John's therapist helps him dissect this thought pattern, asking him to consider the evidence for and against his belief. They explore questions like, "How many times have you actually had a panic attack in these situations?" and "What's the worst that has happened?" Through this, John realizes that, while he has felt anxious, he's never had a panic attack in a meeting, and his fear of judgment is based on assumption rather than fact.

Together, they work on creating a more balanced thought, such as, "Feeling anxious doesn't mean I'll lose control or be judged. I've been anxious before and managed it. Even if I do feel panicked, I have strategies to cope." This new perspective helps John approach previously feared situations with less dread, reducing the intensity and frequency of his panic attacks. Over time, through practicing these cognitive techniques and facing his fears in a controlled manner, John's panic attacks become less frequent, and he feels more confident in his ability to manage his anxiety.

Behavioral techniques, particularly exposure therapy, form another cornerstone of CBT's approach to panic attacks. Exposure therapy involves a gradual and controlled process of facing the feared situations or sensations in a safe and supportive environment. This method helps desensitize individuals to their triggers, reducing the intensity of their panic over time and building confidence in their ability to cope.

Lisa struggles in crowded places. They trigger her panic attacks, leading her to withdraw from social situations. With CBT, Lisa embarks on a journey with her therapist to uncover and challenge the negative thoughts that amplify her fear of crowds. They explore thoughts like, "I'll have a panic attack and embarrass myself" or "I can't handle being in a crowd," evaluating these beliefs and testing their accuracy. Simultaneously, Lisa is gently guided through exposure exercises, starting with visiting a semi-crowded place during off-peak hours, gradually working up to more crowded environments. With each step, Lisa learns practical skills to manage her anxiety, reinforcing her sense of control and diminishing her fear of panic attacks.

Through understanding triggers, restructuring negative thoughts, and applying behavioral techniques, CBT provides a comprehensive framework for individuals to reclaim their lives from the clutches of panic attacks, illustrating the power of this therapeutic approach.

How Can Medications Improve Symptoms of Panic Disorder?

Medications play a pivotal role in managing panic disorder, offering relief from the gripping fear and physical symptoms that characterize this condition. Among the arsenal of treatments, selective serotonin reuptake inhibitors (SSRIs) and benzodiazepines stand out for their effectiveness and mechanisms of action.

SSRIs, such as fluoxetine or sertraline, target the brain's serotonin levels—a key neurotransmitter involved in mood regulation. By preventing the reabsorption (reuptake) of serotonin in the brain, SSRIs increase serotonin availability in the synaptic gap, helping to stabilize mood and reduce anxiety. This adjustment doesn't happen overnight; it usually takes several weeks for SSRIs to build up in the system and exert their full effect. For someone like John, who experiences recurrent panic attacks, starting an SSRI under the careful supervision of a psychiatrist can gradually decrease both the frequency and intensity of his panic attacks. Over time, as the medication helps recalibrate his brain's response to anxiety triggers and CBT helps to expose the underlying thought patterns that lead to anxiety,

John finds that he's facing fewer panic attacks and feeling generally more stable and less anxious in his day-to-day life.

On the other hand, benzodiazepines, including medications like lorazepam or clonazepam, act more quickly and are often utilized for immediate relief during an acute panic episode. These medications work by enhancing the effect of the neurotransmitter GABA (gamma-aminobutyric acid), which inhibits nerve transmission in the brain, leading to a calming effect. During a panic attack, when someone like Lisa feels overwhelmed by sudden intense anxiety and physical symptoms, taking a prescribed benzodiazepine can quickly help to ease these distressing symptoms, providing rapid relief. However, due to their potential for dependence and withdrawal issues, benzodiazepines are generally recommended for short-term use or specific situations where quick intervention is needed.

Both SSRIs and benzodiazepines offer valuable benefits in the treatment of panic disorder, whether for long-term management or immediate relief. The choice between these medications—or the decision to use them in tandem—depends on a person's specific symptoms, treatment history, and overall health profile, highlighting the importance of a personalized approach under professional guidance. Through a combination of these medications, individuals with panic disorder can find significant relief from their symptoms, enabling them to pursue a more calm and fulfilling life.

How Can Regular Physical Activity, Sleep, and a Balanced Diet Improve Symptoms of Panic Disorder?

Managing panic disorder goes beyond traditional therapy and medication; it extends into how we live our daily lives. Incorporating regular physical activity, ensuring adequate sleep, and maintaining a balanced diet can profoundly impact the severity and frequency of panic attacks, providing a more holistic approach to treatment.

Regular exercise is more than just a strategy for physical health; it's a powerful tool for managing anxiety and stress. Engaging in physical activities, such as walking, running, or yoga, triggers the release of endorphins, the body's natural mood lifters. These endorphins can help counteract feelings of anxiety and promote a sense of well-being. Let's look back at John, for example. As part of his ongoing commitment to decreasing the anxiety he feels, he decides to incorporate morning walks into his daily routine. By making daily walks a non-negotiable part of his routine, he boosts his physical health and notices a significant drop in his overall anxiety levels. This reduction in stress contributes to fewer panic attacks, demonstrating how regular exercise can be a key player in managing panic disorder.

Adequate sleep plays a crucial role in emotional regulation and resilience, serving as a foundation for mental well-being. Quality sleep helps the brain process emotional information, recharge, and build defenses against daily stressors. For someone like Lisa, establishing a consistent sleep routine and prioritizing seven to eight hours of sleep each night can lead to notable improvements in mood stability. This consistency in sleep patterns can decrease the occurrence of panic attacks, showing how integral a good night's rest is in the battle against panic disorder.

Similarly, a balanced diet rich in nutrients, supports brain health and emotional stability. Foods high in omega-3 fatty acids, antioxidants, and vitamins nourish the brain and play a role in mood regulation. By incorporating more whole foods, fruits, and vegetables into her diet, energy levels increase and mental well-being improves. This positive change in diet can indirectly help manage panic disorder symptoms by establishing a more stable emotional state and enhancing resilience to stress.

Tackling panic disorder requires a multi-faceted approach that combines psychotherapy and medication with lifestyle adjustments. CBT equips individuals with the tools to navigate panic-inducing thoughts, while medications offer both immediate relief and long-term stability. Beyond these treatments, integrating regular physical activity, adequate sleep, and a balanced diet into one's daily routine can significantly contribute to overall mental well-being. This comprehensive strategy, often developed through collaboration between individuals, therapists, and healthcare professionals, underscores the importance of a personalized and holistic approach to managing panic disorder.

Shedding Light on Social Anxiety Disorder (SAD)

We've all felt nervous or self-conscious in social situations at some point, but for some people, that feeling never goes away. Social anxiety disorder (SAD) is a real, diagnosable mental health condition that affects fifteen million adults, or 6.8 percent of the U.S. population (Anxiety and Depression Association of America, 2020). It's not just a case of being shy or introverted; it's a deeply ingrained fear of being scrutinized or judged by others in social or performance situations. Imagine feeling like you're constantly on stage with the spotlight always shining on you. That's what life can be like for those with SAD. It can have a major impact on a person's life, making it difficult to form relationships, hold down a job, or even leave the house. But with the right treatment and support, it's possible to overcome this debilitating disorder and live a fulfilling life.

SAD can indeed have a profound impact on various aspects of an individual's life, making routine activities challenging due to overwhelming fears of negative judgment or embarrassment. That's why it's important to understand how SAD can affect daily life and the potential consequences over time.

SAD casts a long shadow over the lives of those it touches, infiltrating daily activities and social interactions with a persistent fear of being judged or scrutinized. For someone like John, for whom panic attacks are a symptom of SAD, routine work meetings or casual social gatherings morph into insurmountable challenges. The overwhelming fear of negative evaluation makes these situations intensely uncomfortable and significantly hampers his ability to participate in them, affecting both his professional and personal life.

This fear often leads individuals with SAD down a path of avoidance behavior, a self-protective strategy that ultimately does more harm than good. John, for instance, finds himself dodging group lunches at work, choosing solitude over the anxiety of eating in public. While such avoidance may momentarily reduce anxiety, it also reinforces the fear, trapping him in a cycle of avoidance that limits his experiences and opportunities for social connection.

The repercussions of this avoidance behavior extend deeply into mental health. Constantly sidestepping social interactions can spiral into feelings of isolation, as in an effort to avoid anxiety-provoking situations, the person finds themselves increasingly alone. This isolation can exacerbate the condition, intensifying the sense of being disconnected and misunderstood. Furthermore, the persistent dread of being negatively judged can chip away at one's self-esteem. John's continuous fear of criticism led him to question his worth and abilities, gradually eroding his self-confidence and reinforcing a negative self-image.

Over time, the cumulative effect of these experiences can pave the way for depression. John's story illustrates this progression; what started as a struggle with social anxiety, over time, blossomed into a broader sense of hopelessness, sadness, and a disinterest in life. This highlights the potential for SAD to be a contributing factor to the development of depression.

Understanding social anxiety disorder as a condition that impacts far more than just the ability to mingle at parties is crucial. It's a disorder that can disrupt everyday life, limiting opportunities, straining relationships, and impacting mental health. However, it's not an insurmountable condition. Recognizing the signs early, seeking professional help, and engaging in treatments like cognitive behavioral therapy can open the door to overcoming the fears and challenges posed by SAD. Through gradual exposure to feared situations, support from loved ones, and professional guidance, individuals can reclaim the social aspects of their lives, breaking free from the cycle of avoidance and establishing resilience against the symptoms of social anxiety.

The treatment approach for social anxiety disorder is multifaceted, incorporating various strategies to address both the cognitive and physiological aspects of anxiety. Let's delve into the key components of SAD treatment.

How Can Regular Cognitive Behavioral Therapy (CBT) Improve symptoms of Social Anxiety Disorder?

Regular CBT offers a beacon of hope for those grappling with SAD, presenting a structured and evidence-based pathway to understanding and managing the intense fear of social situations. Otte (2011) systematically reviewed the effectiveness of cognitive behavioral therapy across various anxiety disorders, including SAD, concluding that CBT showed significant benefits in improving symptoms through structured approaches to modifying thought patterns and behaviors.

CBT begins with the meticulous task of unraveling the thought patterns that fuel social anxiety. For many with SAD, distorted beliefs about being scrutinized or judged negatively by others dominate their thought processes, leading to overwhelming anxiety in social settings. CBT guides individuals in identifying these maladaptive thoughts, examining their validity, and challenging their accuracy. This process of cognitive restructuring enables individuals to replace irrational fears with more balanced and realistic perspectives, thereby diminishing the power these thoughts have over their emotional responses.

Another critical component of CBT for SAD is exposure therapy. Just as we saw with panic disorder, this technique is effective for those dealing with SAD because it involves a gradual, controlled approach to confronting feared social situations rather than avoiding them. When individuals are incrementally exposed to the very scenarios they dread, in a supportive and therapeutic context, they can work on becoming desensitized to their triggers of anxiety over time. This method reduces the immediate anxiety response and builds confidence in handling future social interactions.

Through the dual approach of understanding thought patterns and engaging in exposure therapy, regular CBT provides individuals with SAD the tools to navigate social landscapes with increased confidence and less fear. By directly addressing the roots of social anxiety and offering practical strategies for change, CBT stands as a powerful intervention for improving symptoms of social anxiety disorder, paving the way for more fulfilling social interactions and overall well-being.

How Can Medications Improve Symptoms of Social Anxiety Disorder?

Medications are an important aspect of treating SAD, offering those affected a way to manage their symptoms and improve their quality of life. Among the most commonly prescribed medications for SAD are selective serotonin reuptake inhibitors (SSRIs) and beta-blockers, each serving distinct purposes in the management of the disorder.

For those dealing with SAD, SSRIs work in the same way as they do for individuals suffering with panic disorder, targeting the neurotransmitter serotonin in the brain.

Beta-blockers, on the other hand, offer a different approach to managing SAD, particularly its physical symptoms. Medications like propranolol work by blocking the effects of adrenaline, a hormone that plays a significant role in the body's fight-or-flight response. By mitigating adrenaline's impact, beta-blockers can reduce physical symptoms of anxiety such as trembling, sweating, and a rapid heartbeat. This makes them especially useful in specific, anxiety-inducing situations like public speaking.

While SSRIs and beta-blockers serve different aspects of SAD, their use underscores the importance of a tailored treatment plan that addresses both the emotional and physical facets of anxiety. By combining these medications with other treatment modalities, such as CBT, individuals with SAD can find comprehensive support for their condition, paving the way for improved social interaction and overall well-being.

How Can Self-Care Practices Improve Symptoms of Social Anxiety Disorder?

Self-care practices can play a crucial role in managing SAD, offering individuals accessible tools to cope with anxiety in their daily lives. These practices, which include deep breathing, yoga, and progressive muscle relaxation, target both the mind and body, helping to mitigate the symptoms of anxiety that can be so debilitating for those with SAD.

Deep breathing exercises are a simple yet effective technique for calming the nervous system. By focusing on slow, deliberate breaths, individuals can influence their body's response to stress, promoting relaxation and reducing anxiety. For someone like Lisa, who experiences heightened anxiety leading to panic attacks before crowded social events, taking a few minutes to engage in deep breathing can help center her thoughts and diminish her overall anxiety, making social interactions more manageable.

Yoga, with its combination of physical postures, mindfulness, and controlled breathing, offers a holistic approach to anxiety management. By bringing awareness to a connection between mind and body, yoga helps to release physical tension and quiet racing thoughts, both of which are common in SAD. For example, Lisa finds that incorporating regular yoga sessions into her routine enhances her physical well-being and significantly alleviates her social anxiety. The practice encourages her to remain present and grounded, reducing the impact of anxious thoughts.

Progressive muscle relaxation (which will be further detailed in chapter 8) is another technique that can be particularly beneficial for those with SAD. This method involves sequentially tensing and then relaxing different muscle groups throughout the body, which can help to reduce overall tension and anxiety. For Jamie, who we saw earlier suffers from GAD, practicing progressive muscle relaxation before attending social events helps to lower his physical symptoms of anxiety, such as muscle tightness and an accelerated heartbeat, making it easier for him to engage in social situations.

Incorporating self-care practices like deep breathing, yoga, and progressive muscle relaxation into a comprehensive treatment plan for SAD can provide significant benefits. These techniques, alongside psychotherapy and medication, form a multi-faceted approach to managing social anxiety. They empower individuals to take an active role in their treatment, using practical tools to cope with anxiety in everyday situations. Ongoing communication with healthcare professionals is essential, ensuring that each component of the treatment plan is tailored to the individual's needs and adjusted as necessary to support recovery and improve quality of life.

Seasonal Affective Disorder

Have you ever noticed yourself feeling unusually down during the fall or winter months? It's not uncommon to experience a type of depression known as seasonal affective disorder during this time. This sneaky culprit tends to creep in when there is less natural sunlight. This happens because sunlight is necessary for the brain to produce enough serotonin—the neurotransmitter that helps regulate mood—and melatonin, the hormone that helps regulate sleep.

Suddenly you're feeling low energy, like you're constantly moving in slow motion. You may become easily annoyed by others, struggle to focus on everyday tasks, and experience changes in sleep patterns and appetite. Not exactly the recipe for a joyful holiday season. But don't let this disorder keep you from enjoying all the winter fun. There are ways to combat seasonal affective disorder and keep your spirits high!

One effective method is light therapy, which uses a special lamp that mimics natural sunlight to regulate the body's circadian rhythm. Another option is to spend time outdoors during daylight hours or to exercise regularly, which can boost mood and increase energy levels.

I've recently picked up gardening again, something I had always enjoyed but had to give up due to a schedule that demanded most of my attention. The difference I have found in my mood overall is astronomical! This shows how important it is to get our bodies up and about.

Additionally, talking to a therapist or counselor can provide emotional support and help develop coping strategies to manage seasonal affective disorder symptoms. With the right combination of treatments, those who suffer from SAD can still enjoy life, even during the darker winter months.

Some Strategies for Managing Seasonal Affective Disorder

Navigating seasonal affective disorder doesn't have to feel like an uphill battle once you're armed with the right strategies. Given that seasonal affective disorder is closely tied to the ebb and flow of the seasons, particularly the reduced sunlight in winter, finding ways to compensate for that loss is key.

Vitamin D

Vitamin D steps into the spotlight here, especially during those gloomy winter months. Since our bodies usually make vitamin D directly from sunlight, shorter days mean we get less of this mood-boosting nutrient. That's where supplements can make a big difference. Take Jane, for instance. Diagnosed with seasonal affective disorder, she starts taking vitamin D supplements as winter rolls in, aiming to offset the lack of natural light. It's a simple move that supports her mood and overall well-being through the darker days.

Vitamin D's role in mood regulation has been increasingly recognized, with several studies exploring its effects on mental health, including mood disorders like depression and bipolar disorder. A study by Silva et al. (2023) reviewed the literature on vitamin D's role in the evolution and exacerbation of mood disorders, particularly focusing on bipolar affective disorder and depression. The review highlighted vitamin D's functions in suppressing the production of pro-inflammatory cytokines and increasing levels of anti-inflammatory ones, which is relevant given the association of bipolar disorder with increased pro-inflammatory cytokines. Moreover, vitamin D was found to act as an antagonist of glucocorticoids, which are excessively active in mood disorders, and may regulate the formation of new neurons in the hippocampus, underlining its significance in the central nervous system's functioning and immune regulation.

Another study by Murphy and Wagner (2008) conducted an integrative review assessing the association between vitamin D and mood disorders affecting women. The review found that low levels of vitamin D were associated with higher incidences of several mood disorders, including premenstrual syndrome, seasonal affective disorder, non-specified mood disorder, and major depressive disorder, indicating a potential biochemical mechanism between vitamin D and mood disorders in women.

These studies demonstrate the importance of having healthy levels of vitamin D to help regulate our mental health.

Light Therapy

We also have light therapy, a real game-changer for many with seasonal affective disorder. This approach involves soaking up bright, artificial light from a special lamp or lightbox that mimics the sun's rays, tricking your brain into thinking it's still basking in the summer glow. A study by Golden et al. (2005) provides a thorough examination of the effectiveness of light therapy, particularly in treating seasonal affective disorder. The study's primary objective was to evaluate the evidence from randomized controlled trials to determine how effective light therapy is in managing mood disorders, with a specific focus on both seasonal and non-seasonal depression.

To achieve this, the researchers conducted a systematic search of the PubMed database, covering studies from January 1975 to July 2003. They selected only those studies that met rigorous criteria, such as having a control group and using standardized treatment protocols. The selected studies were then analyzed to synthesize their findings.

The results of the meta-analysis revealed that bright light therapy is particularly effective in reducing the severity of symptoms in patients with seasonal affective disorder. The study found that light therapy, especially bright light treatment and dawn simulation, had significant effects comparable to those of antidepressant medications. These findings underscore the potential of light therapy as a first-line treatment for seasonal affective disorder, offering a non-pharmacological alternative that can achieve similar outcomes in symptom reduction. The study also highlighted the importance of using standardized approaches in light therapy to maximize its effectiveness and ensure consistent results across different patient populations.

In essence, while seasonal affective disorder can cast a shadow over the colder months, there are effective ways to fight back. From boosting your vitamin D levels and embracing light therapy to understanding the disorder's seasonal nature, these strategies offer a beacon of hope. And remember, it's always a good idea to discuss these options with a healthcare professional to tailor the approach to your needs. With the right plan in place, winter doesn't have to be so bleak after all.

Obsessive-Compulsive Disorder (OCD)

Have you ever found yourself double-checking if you turned off the stove or washing your hands repeatedly, even though you know you already did it? This may just be a quirk for some, but for others, it can be a sign of obsessive-compulsive disorder. OCD is a mental health disorder that causes persistent, intrusive thoughts or obsessions that lead to repetitive behaviors or compulsions. These compulsions are done in an attempt to alleviate the anxiety associated with the obsessions. The themes of the obsessions can vary widely, from fear of contamination to fear of making a mistake. The compulsions can also vary, from checking to counting, and even seeking reassurance. It's important to seek help if you or someone you know is struggling with OCD, as it can greatly impact daily life. OCD can affect people of all ages, and often starts in childhood or adolescence.

According to the *Diagnostic and Statistical Manual of Mental Disorders 5th Edition* (*DSM-5*), some of the common symptoms of OCD include the presence of obsessions, compulsions, or both. Obsessions are often described as persistent, intrusive, and unwanted thoughts, urges, or mental images that cause significant distress or anxiety. Compulsions, on the other hand, refer to repetitive and ritualistic behaviors or mental acts that an individual performs in response to their obsessions.

OCD patients experience recurrent and persistent thoughts, images, or impulses that are intrusive and cause anxiety or distress. To cope with this anxiety, individuals with OCD engage in repetitive behaviors or mental acts aimed at reducing anxiety, often without any logical explanation or sense. For example, a person with OCD may repeatedly check if they have locked the door, even though they already know they did. This behavior can take up a significant amount of time and interfere with daily activities, leaving individuals feeling anxious, drained, and isolated.

While symptoms may fluctuate in intensity over time, the disorder can significantly interfere with daily functioning, relationships, and overall quality of life. Unfortunately, OCD commonly co-occurs with other mental health disorders, such as depression, anxiety disorders, and eating disorders, making it even more challenging to manage. Despite the significant challenges that come with OCD, with support and effective treatment, individuals can manage their symptoms and improve their quality of life.

Cognitive Behavioral Therapy's Role in Treating OCD

Fortunately, CBT can prove highly effective in managing these symptoms. One popular technique within CBT is called exposure and response prevention (ERP). This approach involves confronting one's irrational fears or obsessions (exposure) and refraining from engaging in compulsive, anxiety-reducing behaviors (response prevention).

How ERP Works

The process of ERP involves a series of steps that gradually expose you to your fears without giving in to compulsions, helping you learn to tolerate anxiety and reduce obsessive behaviors over time.

The journey begins with the essential step of recognizing and understanding your obsessions. It's about identifying those intrusive thoughts or fears that cause distress and disrupt your life. For example, someone might be overwhelmed by the fear of contamination, constantly worrying about germs. Once these obsessions are recognized, the next crucial step is partnering with a therapist who specializes in CBT for OCD. This collaboration is the cornerstone of your treatment, providing the guidance and support needed as you navigate the complexities of therapy.

Together with your therapist, you'll develop a hierarchy of fears—a list of situations that trigger your anxiety, ranked from least to most distressing. This hierarchy serves as your guide for exposure exercises. You'll start with situations that provoke the least anxiety, gradually exposing yourself to these triggers. For instance, if contamination is your fear, you might begin by touching something you consider only slightly contaminated, resisting the urge to immediately wash your hands. During these exposures, it's crucial to stay present, practicing mindfulness to tolerate the discomfort without resorting to compulsive behaviors.

Keeping a journal throughout this process is invaluable. It helps you track your experiences, monitor your anxiety levels, and reflect on the outcomes, revealing the irrationality of your fears over time. As you become more comfortable with lower levels of anxiety, you'll gradually move up your hierarchy, facing more challenging exposures. This steady progression is key to desensitizing yourself to the stimuli that once controlled you.

Through ERP and other proven CBT techniques, people with OCD can gain control over their anxiety and depression, leading to a more fulfilling and peaceful life overall.

Post-Traumatic Stress Disorder (PTSD)

Post-traumatic stress disorder (PTSD) is a serious mental health condition that can impact anyone who has experienced or witnessed a traumatic event. It's not uncommon for people who have gone through a traumatic experience to struggle to cope with their emotions and memories afterward, and PTSD is one of the conditions that can develop as a result.

Whether it's a single traumatic incident or prolonged exposure to distressing events, PTSD can be a life-changing struggle that requires professional help to overcome. While PTSD can develop for a variety of reasons, some of the most common causes include war, combat, sexual assault, natural disasters, accidents, or witnessing violence. It's important for anyone who is experiencing symptoms consistent with PTSD to seek help and support as soon as possible to prevent the condition from worsening.

Understanding PTSD is essential for recognizing its impact and navigating the path to recovery. Its symptoms are multifaceted, often profoundly influencing one's emotional state, thought processes, and overall ability to function.

PTSD often also manifests through re-experiencing symptoms, such as flashbacks, intrusive memories, and nightmares, which are hallmark signs of the disorder. These distressing recollections force individuals to relive their trauma repeatedly, disrupting daily life and causing significant emotional turmoil. Alongside this, avoidance behaviors are common. Individuals may go to great lengths to avoid anything that reminds them of the trauma, whether it's specific places, activities, or even certain thoughts and conversations that could trigger painful memories.

The disorder also brings about profound negative changes in mood and cognition. Those affected may develop persistent negative beliefs about themselves or view the world through a lens of mistrust and danger. This altered perception often causes deep feelings of guilt, shame, and alienation, which can erode a sense of self and strain relationships with others.

Arousal and reactivity symptoms, like hypervigilance, irritability, and an exaggerated startle response, reflect the body's constant state of heightened alertness, making it difficult to relax or feel secure. Sleep disturbances, including trouble falling or staying asleep, further intensify this state of unease, taking a toll on physical health and emotional resilience.

For a PTSD diagnosis, these symptoms must persist for more than a month and significantly impair daily functioning. Interestingly, symptoms can sometimes be delayed, emerging months or even years after the traumatic event, complicating both diagnosis and treatment.

The impact of PTSD extends beyond the individual, often impairing relationships and work life. Trust issues, emotional numbing, and withdrawal can make it challenging to maintain close connections or perform effectively at work. Furthermore, PTSD rarely occurs in isolation; it frequently coexists with other mental health conditions like depression, anxiety, and substance abuse, creating a complex web of psychological challenges.

Some Therapeutic Techniques for Managing PTSD

Recognizing the symptoms of PTSD and understanding their impact is a crucial first step toward seeking help. Effective treatment for PTSD often involves a combination of psychotherapy and medication. Psychotherapy techniques such as cognitive behavioral therapy and Eye Movement Desensitization and Reprocessing (EMDR) are commonly used, alongside medications to help manage symptoms. Early intervention and support from mental health professionals can significantly improve outcomes, helping individuals regain control over their lives from the grip of trauma.

Cognitive Behavioral Therapy's Impact on PTSD

CBT is a cornerstone in treating PTSD, offering various techniques to help individuals manage their symptoms. Two of the most effective methods within CBT are prolonged exposure (PE) and Eye Movement Desensitization and Reprocessing (EMDR), each providing unique ways to address PTSD.

PE focuses on helping individuals confront their fears directly. The idea is that by gradually facing trauma-related situations or memories, people can learn to tolerate and process the intense emotions associated with them. For example, consider Michael, who avoids anything that reminds him of his traumatic experience. In PE, Michael would first learn relaxation techniques to help him manage anxiety. Then, he and his therapist would create a list of situations that he fears, starting with those that provoke the least anxiety. Over time, Michael would be guided through these situations, helping him to stay present and resist the urge to avoid them. This controlled exposure gradually reduces the power these triggers have over him, decreasing his PTSD symptoms.

On the other hand, EMDR combines recalling traumatic memories with a specific type of distraction, such as following the therapist's finger with your eyes. This technique helps the brain reprocess traumatic memories, making them less emotionally overwhelming. For instance, Hannah, who feels consumed by traumatic memories, might focus on a particularly distressing event while following the therapist's finger back and forth. This dual focus is believed to help her brain integrate and reprocess the traumatic memory, reducing its emotional intensity.

Both PE and EMDR demonstrate the versatility and effectiveness of CBT in treating PTSD. These structured, step-by-step approaches empower individuals to face and reframe their traumatic experiences, leading to substantial improvements in their daily lives.

In addition to psychotherapy, medications, particularly SSRIs, are often used to help manage PTSD symptoms. SSRIs can help stabilize mood and reduce symptoms of depression and anxiety that frequently accompany PTSD. It's essential, however, that any medication is carefully monitored by a healthcare professional and tailored to the individual's specific needs.

Combining therapeutic techniques like PE and EMDR with appropriate medication represents a comprehensive approach to managing PTSD. This integrated strategy addresses the complex nature of PTSD, ensuring that individuals receive the most effective treatment tailored to their unique symptoms and experiences.

3

STRESS LESS: OVERCOMING THE INVISIBLE ENEMY

Stress is often seen as an invisible enemy that creeps up on us when we least expect it. It can lead to anxiety and depression, which can have a profound impact on our mental health. However, by understanding the nature of stress and how it relates to these other mental health conditions, we can take steps to manage it more effectively. Whether it's meditation, exercise, or talking to a therapist, there are numerous strategies we can employ to reduce stress and improve our overall well-being. In chapter 3 we'll explore how to stress less and overcome the invisible enemy so that we can take control of our mental health and live a happier, more fulfilling life.

Stress: the Good, the Bad, and the Ugly

The word "stress" often conjures up negative emotions, but did you know that sometimes it can be a good thing? When we experience stress in small amounts, it can actually help us perform better and achieve our goals. For example, a looming deadline can motivate us to work harder and be more productive, resulting in better work quality. And when it comes to athletics, many athletes thrive under pressure, using the added stress to give them an extra boost of energy and determination.

However, the effects of chronic stress on our health cannot be overstated. While we all experience stress at some point in our lives, chronic stress can lead to serious physical and mental health issues. It's not surprising that many people who suffer from anxiety and depression also have high levels of chronic stress. Strong scientific evidence now suggests that chronic stress can be a significant contributing factor to the development of anxiety and depression (Yaribeygi et al., 2017). The body's natural stress response system, once activated repeatedly over prolonged periods of time, can lead to imbalances in certain chemicals within the brain, ultimately leading to chronic anxiety or depression.

The symptoms of chronic stress are numerous, ranging from physical symptoms like headaches and difficulty sleeping to emotional symptoms like irritability and worry. These symptoms can be overwhelming, affecting every aspect of our lives. If left untreated, chronic stress can have serious long-term consequences on our well-being. Studies have shown that chronic stress can cause structural changes in the brain, particularly in the areas responsible for memory and mood regulation (Saeedi and Rashiday-Pour, 2021). Researchers have also found that chronic stress can cause a decrease in the size of the hippocampus, which is the area of the brain that plays a crucial role in memory and learning. This structural change can result in cognitive impairment, making it difficult to learn and remember new things.

The first step to stress management is recognizing the signs of stress and understanding its nature. Knowing these warning signs can help you take steps to reduce stress before it becomes too overwhelming.

Additionally, understanding how stress contributes to anxiety and depression can motivate you to take stress management seriously and seek out strategies to prevent it. Overall, taking control of your stress can help you feel happier, more productive, and more fulfilled in your daily life.

The Stress Response: Fight or Flight

When you're faced with a stressful situation, your body goes into fight-or-flight mode. This is an ancient survival mechanism designed to help you either confront the danger or run away from it. Your body releases stress hormones like adrenaline and cortisol, which increase your heart rate, sharpen your senses, and prepare your muscles for action. Once the threat passes, your body is supposed to return to a state of calm.

But in today's world, stress isn't usually about escaping from predators. It's more about dealing with work pressures, financial worries, or relationship problems, challenges that don't go away easily. When stress becomes a constant in your life, your body stays in a heightened state of alert, which can lead to a range of physical and mental health issues, including anxiety and depression.

Stress and Anxiety: a Vicious Cycle

Stress and anxiety are closely linked. When you're stressed, your body is on high alert, and this can make you feel anxious. On the flip side, if you're already prone to anxiety, stressful situations can make your anxiety symptoms worse. It's a bit of a vicious cycle—stress increases anxiety, and anxiety makes it harder to deal with stress.

Let's look at some examples that showcase how chronic stress can lead to anxiety. For instance, Sarah, who has been working in a high-stress corporate job for over a decade, starts to experience symptoms of anxiety and depression. She begins having panic attacks at work, constantly feels overwhelmed with worry, struggles to sleep at night, and loses interest in activities she once loved, like hiking and reading. Similarly, David, a college student, has been under immense academic pressure throughout his studies. The constant demand to maintain high grades, meet the expectations of his family, and the fear of failure starts to take a toll on him. He begins to feel anxious before every exam, withdraws from social activities, and feels hopeless about his future.

Stress and Depression: the Weight of the World

Chronic stress doesn't just fuel anxiety, it can also lead to depression. When you're stressed, your body is constantly producing cortisol, the stress hormone. While cortisol is helpful in short bursts, prolonged exposure to high levels of cortisol can lead to changes in your brain chemistry, making you more susceptible to depression.

Stress can also contribute to feelings of helplessness or hopelessness, which are key symptoms of depression. If you're dealing with ongoing stress at work and feel like there's no way out, you might start to feel trapped and overwhelmed. Over time, these feelings can turn into depression, making it hard to find joy in anything or motivate yourself to make positive changes.

Understanding the connection between stress, anxiety, and depression is the first step in breaking the cycle. By recognizing how stress contributes to anxiety and depression, you can take steps to manage it more effectively, helping to protect your mental health and improve your overall well-being. Here are some strategies to help manage stress and protect your mental health.

Breaking the Cycle: Managing Stress to Improve Mental Health

Life can feel like a never-ending whirlwind, with stress weaving its way into our daily lives. But here's the good news: you can break the cycle and take control of your mental health with a few effective strategies. Let's explore some fun and engaging ways to keep stress in check while boosting your overall well-being.

Embrace Physical Activity: Move Your Way to Better Mood

Exercise isn't just about staying fit; it's also a natural mood booster. When you move, your body releases endorphins, those feel-good hormones that help combat stress and anxiety.

Pick activities that you genuinely enjoy. Whether it's the calming flow of yoga, the energetic beats of a dance class, or the refreshing splash of swimming, doing what you love makes it easier to stick with it.

The Magic of a Simple Walk

Never underestimate the power of a stroll! A study from the *Journal of Happiness Studies* in 2018 highlighted how even a short walk in nature can lift your spirits and reduce stress. So lace up those shoes and get walking!

Dance Away Stress: Let the Rhythm Move You

Dancing isn't just exercise; it's also a fun, expressive way to release stress. Whether you're grooving in your living room or hitting the dance floor, letting loose can be incredibly liberating. Pair your moves with music that resonates with your mood. Create a playlist that makes you want to dance your heart out, letting the rhythm guide you to a happier state of mind.

Dive into Serenity: the Soothing Power of Swimming

Swimming offers a unique sense of calm. The water's gentle resistance, combined with the rhythmic strokes, creates a meditative environment that helps melt away stress. While you swim, focus on each movement and the sensation of the water. This turns your swim into a mindful practice that soothes both body and mind.

Crafting Calm: How Your Environment Can Reduce Stress

Your surroundings play a huge role in how you feel. Just like the right music can set the mood, creating a calm and serene environment can help melt away stress and bring more peace into your life. Let's dive into some simple yet powerful ways to turn your space into a sanctuary of tranquility.

Declutter for Peace of Mind (Clear Space, Clear Mind)

Clutter can make us feel overwhelmed and stressed. By decluttering, you create a more organized and serene space, which helps clear your mind as well, giving your surroundings and your thoughts a little breathing room. Start by simplifying your spaces. Organize your belongings so everything has its place, and keep only what truly adds value or joy to your life. A tidy space leads to a tidier mind, helping you feel more in control and less stressed.

Bring the Outdoors In: the Power of Indoor Plants

Indoor plants aren't just pretty; they're also great for your mental health. Adding greenery to your space can reduce stress and boost your mood, contributing to a sense of calm and well-being. Plants like succulents, ferns, and peace lilies are low-maintenance options that bring a touch of nature indoors. Turn your home or workspace into a mini green oasis. Even a small plant on your desk or a few potted herbs in the kitchen can make a difference.

Light and Space: Designing for Tranquility

Natural light is a natural mood lifter. Make sure your living and working spaces are well-lit with sunlight during the day. Light helps improve your mood and creates a warm and inviting atmosphere. An uncluttered, open space can feel freeing and calm. Arrange your furniture to allow for easy movement and keep your rooms airy. This openness can create a sense of peace and help you feel more relaxed.

The Colors of Calm

Colors have a powerful impact on our emotions. Soft blues, greens, and neutral tones can evoke a sense of calm and serenity. Use these colors in your decor to create a peaceful environment that helps you unwind. Lighting sets the mood in a room. Opt for soft, warm-toned lighting that creates a cozy and tranquil ambiance. Lamps with dimmers or warm bulbs can turn any room into a relaxing retreat.

The Power of Connection: Social Support as a Stress Reliever

One of the most effective ways to combat stress is through connection with others. Spending quality time with friends and family can help you feel supported and less anxious. Even a quick phone call during a busy day can provide comfort and ease your mind. Beyond close relationships, being part of a community—whether it's a club, group, or organization—can also be incredibly beneficial. It gives you the chance to meet new people, share experiences, and develop common interests. Human connections are essential for our well-being, so make time to nurture these bonds and watch your stress levels decrease. By thoughtfully designing your environment, prioritizing sleep, and staying connected with others, you can create a life that's not just less stressful, but filled with moments of calm and joy.

When to Seek Professional Help

Stress is an inevitable part of life, but when it starts to take control of your thoughts and actions, seeking professional help may be necessary. It's not a sign of weakness to ask for help, but rather a courageous step toward self-care. Chronic feelings of hopelessness or the inability to function in your daily activities due to stress are major warning signs that professional help is needed. Mental health professionals are equipped with the necessary skills to help you manage stress, anxiety, and depression. Remember, taking care of your mental health is just as important as your physical health.

Life can get overwhelming sometimes, and when the stress, anxiety, or feelings of depression start to weigh you down, it's important to recognize when you need a little extra help. Here are some signs that it might be time to reach out to a professional:

- **Stress That Won't Quit.** If stress is hanging around like an unwelcome guest, making it tough to enjoy your day-to-day life, it might be time to talk to someone who can help lighten the load.

- **Persistent Feelings of Hopelessness.** When hopelessness starts to feel like a permanent state of mind, it's more than just a rough patch. A mental health professional can help you find new ways to see the light at the end of the tunnel.

- **Daily Life Is Getting Harder.** If stress or anxiety is making it difficult to keep up with work, relationships, or even basic tasks, it's a strong sign that professional support could be beneficial.

Why Seek Professional Help?

Talking to a psychologist, psychiatrist, or therapist is like getting expert advice for your emotional health. Here's how they can make a big difference:

- **Tailored Strategies Just for You.** Professionals work with you to develop strategies that fit your specific situation. They help you address the root causes of your stress and teach you effective ways to cope.

- **Expert Coping Skills.** With their specialized training, mental health professionals are skilled at equipping you with tools to handle anxiety and depression. They offer you a personalized toolkit for navigating life's challenges. Always remember that reaching out is the bravest step you can take to safeguard your own mental health. Asking for help isn't a sign of weakness; it's a smart and empowering move to improve your mental health. Professionals are there to support you every step of the way. Don't try to handle everything alone; reach out and let the experts guide you toward a healthier, happier version of yourself.

Embracing Support for Your Mental Well-being

To find in-person therapists, check out local mental health clinics, community centers, or university counseling services. Your primary care doctor can also provide recommendations tailored to your situation.

Life can be busy, and sometimes getting to an in-person session isn't easy. Many professionals now offer teletherapy, allowing you to receive support from the comfort of your own home. It's a flexible option that fits into your schedule.

Websites like Psychology Today and Zocdoc are great places to start. They offer detailed profiles of mental health professionals in your area, helping you find the right fit for your needs.

When choosing a mental health professional, consider their specialty, treatment approach, and what past clients have said about them. It's important to find someone who really gets what you're going through.

Check your insurance for mental health coverage, and look for professionals who offer flexible payment options. Some may offer sliding-scale fees or more affordable rates, making support accessible to everyone.

Your well-being is worth prioritizing. Seeking help is a powerful step toward a better, more balanced life. Whether online or in-person, support is available and within reach.

4

A Closer Look at Medication: the Good, the Bad, and the Necessary

I feel like, at some point in life, everyone struggles with the thought of taking medication, especially if it's for something they can't even see. Your own mind gaslights you into thinking that there's nothing wrong with you, and yet it's the same mind tearing your life apart. Sounds morbid, doesn't it?

If you're someone who's had to deal with anxiety and depression, you know that even finding the right medication can be a journey. Sometimes it may feel like you're taking a shot in the dark, trying medication after medication until something finally works. It's not an easy process, but it's worth it to find relief from symptoms that can be debilitating.

In chapter 4 we'll be taking a closer look at medications for anxiety and depression. We'll explore the benefits, possible side effects, and everything in between. By the end, you'll have a better understanding of what's out there to help manage your symptoms, and hopefully, you'll feel empowered to take control of your own treatment journey. So, let's dive in and uncover the good, the bad, and the necessary.

Medications: More than Just a Prescription

It's important to understand that medications for anxiety and depression are not a cure-all. While they can be effective in managing symptoms, they should always be used in conjunction with other forms of therapy. In fact, a combination of medication and therapy has been found to be more effective than medication alone.

A study aimed at comparing the effectiveness of behavioral activation, cognitive therapy, and antidepressant medication in treating major depressive disorder in adults revealed some compelling insights. The research found that for individuals with severe depression, behavioral activation was just as effective as antidepressant medication, and both approaches outperformed cognitive therapy alone. This highlights the importance of integrating multiple therapeutic approaches when treating depression, particularly for those with more intense symptoms, as a combination of treatments can provide the most comprehensive benefit (Dimidjian et al., 2006).

When it comes to medication, it's crucial to remember that side effects can vary significantly from one person to another. While some people might only experience mild issues like nausea or dizziness, others could face more severe effects, such as weight gain or sexual dysfunction. It's essential to communicate openly with your doctor about any side effects you experience so you can work together to adjust your treatment plan as needed.

Another important point is that medication often requires time to show its full benefits. Many antidepressants, including popular options like Lexapro, Zoloft, and Prozac, may take several weeks or even months to take full effect. It's important to stay patient and continue following your prescribed regimen, even if you don't see immediate results. Medications can be highly effective in managing symptoms of anxiety and depression, but they work best when combined with other forms of therapy. Collaborating closely with your healthcare provider to find the most suitable treatment plan is key, and persistence is crucial in achieving the best possible outcome.

Unwrapping the Good: Benefits of Medication

Medications play a crucial role in the treatment of anxiety and depression, often proving to be highly effective in reducing symptoms for many patients. A comprehensive study by Bandelow et al. (2015) analyzed data from numerous randomized controlled trials involving over 37,000 patients, comparing the efficacy of pharmacological, psychological, and combined treatments for major anxiety disorders, including panic disorder, generalized anxiety disorder, and social phobia. The findings revealed that medications had a significantly higher average effect size than psychotherapies alone, indicating their substantial impact in alleviating symptoms across a broad range of patients. This study highlighted the effectiveness of various medications, including serotonin-norepinephrine reuptake inhibitors (SNRIs), benzodiazepines, selective serotonin reuptake inhibitors (SSRIs), and tricyclic antidepressants, underscoring the importance of pharmacological treatment in managing anxiety disorders effectively (Bandelow et al., 2015).

The advantages of medication are multifaceted. For one, medication can significantly reduce the severity of symptoms, enabling individuals to function more effectively in their daily lives. For example, someone experiencing severe panic attacks may find relief with benzodiazepines like Xanax, allowing them to manage their symptoms more effectively. For someone experiencing severe depression, Wellbutrin, an antidepressant commonly prescribed to alleviate symptoms of depression, can be very effective. It belongs to a class of medications known as selective norepinephrine and dopamine reuptake inhibitors (NDRIs). These medications work by increasing the levels of specific neurotransmitters in the brain, such as norepinephrine and dopamine, which are crucial in regulating mood and emotions. By stabilizing these neurotransmitters, Wellbutrin helps create a more manageable emotional state, enabling individuals to engage more effectively in other forms of treatment like psychotherapy.

Medication can also lower the risk of relapse, particularly when used as part of a comprehensive treatment plan that includes therapy and lifestyle changes. In this way, medication becomes a powerful tool in helping individuals manage their anxiety and depression, leading to a better quality of life.

However, it's important to recognize that medication is not a one-size-fits-all solution. Different people may respond better to different types of medication, and it can take some trial and error to find the right fit. Additionally, potential side effects are a critical consideration. Common side effects of antidepressants include nausea, weight gain, and sexual dysfunction. Despite these possible downsides, many patients find that the benefits of medication—such as improved mood and reduced anxiety—far outweigh the risks.

Combining medication with psychotherapy, such as CBT, often proves highly effective for many individuals. While medications like Wellbutrin address the biological aspects of mental health conditions, therapy provides the tools and strategies to manage thoughts, emotions, and behaviors. This dual approach is particularly powerful, as it allows individuals to tackle both the physical and psychological components of their condition. A patient taking Wellbutrin may find it easier to engage in CBT, where they can learn to identify and challenge negative thought patterns and develop healthier behaviors.

Similarly, combining medications like Xanax (alprazolam), commonly prescribed for anxiety, with CBT offers a holistic approach to treating coexisting anxiety and depression. A patient like John, who we saw earlier struggles with severe panic attacks, is more able to engage in CBT while taking Xanax. This is due to Xanax's enhancement on the effects of gamma-aminobutyric acid (GABA) in the brain, providing a calming effect that can significantly reduce anxiety symptoms. This reduction in anxiety can be especially beneficial for those whose depression is aggravated by high anxiety levels, allowing them to engage more fully in therapeutic processes. This integrated treatment approach effectively manages the immediate symptoms of anxiety with medications like Xanax, while addressing the deeper cognitive and behavioral patterns associated with depression through cognitive-behavioral therapy. Close collaboration and regular monitoring between the therapist and prescribing healthcare provider are crucial for evaluating the treatment's progress and making necessary adjustments. This ensures that the strategy remains personalized and effective in improving mental health.

It's important to remember that each treatment plan should be tailored to your unique circumstances. Decisions about medication should always be made in consultation with a qualified healthcare professional, ensuring that the combination of medication and therapy is customized to meet your specific needs and preferences for the best possible outcomes.

Commonly Prescribed Medications

Benzodiazepines: a class of drugs used for decades, these are commonly prescribed to treat anxiety, insomnia, and related disorders. These medications can be highly effective in managing symptoms, helping people lead more productive lives. However, they also come with some risks and potential side effects. Benzodiazepines can be addictive and may cause drowsiness, confusion, and memory problems in some individuals. Because of these risks, it's crucial to work closely with a healthcare provider to ensure the proper dosage and monitoring of symptoms. While benzodiazepines can be beneficial for many, it's important to weigh the benefits against the potential drawbacks when considering any medication.

Examples of Benzodiazepines:
- Alprazolam (Xanax)

- Diazepam (Valium)

- Lorazepam (Ativan)

- Clonazepam (Klonopin)

- Triazolam (Halcion)

Selective Serotonin Reuptake Inhibitors: SSRIs have revolutionized the treatment of depression and anxiety disorders. These medications work by increasing the levels of serotonin in the brain, a neurotransmitter that plays a key role in regulating mood, appetite, and sleep. SSRIs are favored for their relatively fewer side effects and lower toxicity, making them safer for long-term use. They are commonly prescribed for conditions such as major depressive disorder, obsessive-compulsive disorder, and post-traumatic stress disorder, helping countless people regain control over their lives.

Examples of SSRIs:
- Fluoxetine (Prozac)

- Sertraline (Zoloft)

- Paroxetine (Paxil)

- Escitalopram (Lexapro)

- Citalopram (Celexa)

Serotonin-Norepinephrine Reuptake Inhibitors: SNRIs are another class of antidepressants that have gained popularity. SNRIs increase levels of both serotonin and norepinephrine, neurotransmitters involved in mood regulation and emotional stability. This dual action can lead to better outcomes for patients with conditions like depression, anxiety, and

ADHD. SNRIs may be a good option for those seeking an alternative to other antidepressants.

Examples of SNRIs:
- Venlafaxine (Effexor)

- Duloxetine (Cymbalta)

- Desvenlafaxine (Pristiq)

- Levomilnacipran (Fetzima)

Norepinephrine and Dopamine Reuptake Inhibitors: NDRIs are used to treat mental health conditions such as depression, ADHD, and anxiety. NDRIs work by increasing the levels of norepinephrine and dopamine, neurotransmitters that are key to emotional regulation, motivation, and attention. Many patients prefer NDRIs because they often have fewer side effects and can improve overall cognitive function.

Example of NDRI:
- Bupropion (Wellbutrin)

Tricyclic Antidepressants: TCAs have been around for decades and remain a treatment option for depression. Unlike newer antidepressants, TCAs block the reabsorption of both serotonin and norepinephrine, increasing their levels in the brain. While effective, TCAs can come with side effects such as dry mouth, constipation, and blurred vision. However, many people find the benefits in mood and emotional stability outweigh these drawbacks.

Examples of TCAs:
- Amitriptyline (Elavil)

- Imipramine (Tofranil)

- Nortriptyline (Pamelor)

- Clomipramine (Anafranil) - approved for OCD

- Doxepin (Silenor)

- Amoxapine (Asendin)

- Desipramine (Norpramin)

- Protriptyline (Vivactil)

- Trimipramine (Surmontil)

Monoamine Oxidase Inhibitors: MAOIs are a class of medications used to treat various mental health conditions. MAOIs work by inhibiting the enzyme monoamine oxidase, which breaks down neurotransmitters like serotonin and dopamine. By preventing this breakdown, MAOIs can help alleviate symptoms of depression and anxiety. However, they require careful monitoring due to potential interactions with certain foods and other medications.

Examples of MAOIs:
- Phenelzine (Nardil)

- Tranylcypromine (Parnate)

- Isocarboxazid (Marplan)

- Selegiline (Emsam)

Beta-Blockers: these medications are primarily used to treat cardiovascular conditions like hypertension and heart failure by blocking the effects of adrenaline. Recently, they have also been investigated for treating anxiety and migraine headaches. While effective, beta-blockers can cause side effects such as fatigue and dizziness, so they should be used under a healthcare provider's supervision.

Examples of Beta-blockers:

- Propranolol (Inderal)

- Atenolol (Tenormin)

Buspirone is also gaining attention for its potential benefits in treating anxiety disorders. Unlike other anxiety medications, buspirone is not addictive and does not cause drowsiness or memory impairment. It works by increasing serotonin and reducing dopamine levels in the brain. While it may take a few weeks to see its full effects, buspirone is effective in reducing symptoms like excessive worry and tension.

Hydroxyzine, often used to treat allergies, itching, and sleep disorders, also possesses anxiolytic properties. Its sedative and calming effects make it a popular choice for people with anxiety disorders, tackling both physical and psychological symptoms.

Pregabalin, known as Lyrica, was initially developed to treat neuropathic pain but has since been found effective for generalized anxiety disorder. It offers an alternative to traditional anxiety medications, reducing symptoms like constant worry and physical manifestations of anxiety.

This comprehensive overview of different classes of medications highlights the importance of working closely with a healthcare provider to find the most suitable treatment plan tailored to your specific needs and conditions.

The Dark Side: Potential Side Effects

We've all seen those medication commercials with the long lists of side effects recited at lightning speed. When it comes to medication, it is important to remember that while they can provide relief, they can also bring about unwanted side effects. The potential dark side of medication cannot be ignored. From nausea to weight gain and even changes in sleep patterns, medication side effects can be frustrating and sometimes even debilitating.

It's important to talk to your doctor about all potential side effects before starting a new medication and to be vigilant in monitoring any changes you may experience while taking it. While the benefits of medication can be life-changing, the potential negative effects should always be considered.

When it comes to taking medication for mental health issues, one side effect that often flies under the radar is weight gain. For example, Paxil, an antidepressant, is well-known for causing significant weight gain in some people. But weight gain is just one of many potential side effects. Some antidepressants, particularly in the early stages of treatment, may be linked to an increased risk of suicidal thoughts or behaviors, especially in young adults. This risk is generally highest during the first few weeks of treatment, making close monitoring by a healthcare provider essential during this period. This is why it's so important to work closely with a healthcare provider to monitor and manage any side effects, and to find a medication that's right for you. Your mental health is worth the extra care and attention.

Everyone responds differently to medications; what works well for one person might not work as effectively for another, or might cause different side effects. This underscores the importance of personalized treatment plans that take into account your medical history, lifestyle, and other individual factors. Ongoing communication with your healthcare provider is key. If you notice any side effects, whether it's weight gain, mood changes, or anything else, it's important to discuss these concerns as soon as possible. Your provider can adjust your treatment plan, including changing the medication or its dosage, to better fit your needs.

Deciding to take medication, choosing the right one, and finding the correct dosage involves carefully balancing the potential benefits and risks.

This is a collaborative process between you and your healthcare provider, aimed at finding the most effective treatment with the fewest side effects.

In summary, managing psychiatric medications is all about partnership. Regular monitoring, open communication, and flexibility in treatment are all key to success. Additionally, incorporating healthy lifestyle habits like diet and exercise can help manage side effects such as weight gain, making your overall treatment plan more effective and sustainable.

Navigating the Sea of Medication: Making Informed Decisions

When it comes to medication, it's crucial to make informed decisions that take into account both the benefits and drawbacks of different treatments. Fortunately, there are many resources available to help you better understand your medications and make informed choices.

It's crucial to understand both the benefits and potential drawbacks of any medication you are considering for your condition. This includes being aware of possible side effects, interactions with other medications, and any long-term considerations.

Websites like MedlinePlus and Mayo Clinic are excellent resources for accurate and up-to-date information on medications. These sites provide detailed insights into medication uses, dosages, side effects, and precautions. Relying on such reputable sources ensures you are making informed decisions based on solid evidence, rather than anecdotal advice or unreliable information.

Just as finding sources for accurate and reliable information about medications is important, so is finding a trustworthy healthcare provider. Websites like Healthgrades or Zocdoc are useful for finding healthcare providers in your area. These platforms offer patient reviews and detailed information about a provider's background and specialties.

Many healthcare providers now also offer telehealth services, making it easier and more convenient to connect with professionals who can address your mental health needs from the comfort of your home.

Maintaining open communication with your healthcare provider is essential. Your provider can offer personalized guidance tailored to your health history, current medications, and specific needs. It's important to ask questions about the purpose of the medication, potential side effects, and how it fits into your overall treatment plan. This dialogue helps ensure that you fully understand your treatment and feel confident in the decisions being made.

Never hesitate to ask questions if something is unclear. Understanding how a medication works, what side effects to watch for, and how long it might take to see results can help you feel more in control and improve your commitment to the treatment plan.

Finding the right medication can sometimes be a process of trial and error. Not everyone reacts the same way to a given medication, and it may take time to find the one that works best for you with the fewest side effects. Patience is key, and your healthcare provider will support you throughout this journey, making adjustments as needed to find the most effective treatment.

Beyond the Pill: Managing Side Effects and Maximizing Benefits

Managing the side effects of medication can be a challenging task for many patients. In order to ensure you are taking full advantage of your medication while minimizing the negative side effects, it is essential to adopt a holistic approach to treatment. This involves taking medication as prescribed, and taking measures to improve your overall health and well-being.

One of the most effective ways to manage common side effects such as weight gain is through regular exercise and a balanced diet. For example, walking for just thirty minutes each day can help to prevent the weight gain that often accompanies medications such as Remeron. In addition, eating a balanced diet rich in fruits, vegetables, and whole grains can help to counteract any unwanted weight gain.

Regular physical exercise and a balanced diet have been proven through research and studies to have profound benefits on overall health and well-being, including weight management. A study by Snel et al. (2012) looked at how adding exercise to a very low-calorie diet affects people with obesity and type 2 diabetes. Participants were split into two groups: one followed just the diet, while the other combined the diet with regular exercise. Both groups lost a significant amount of weight, but the group that also exercised lost more fat. Additionally, the exercise group showed improvements in muscle health and fitness that the diet-only group didn't. Both groups improved their body's ability to manage insulin, but the added benefits in fat loss and fitness suggest that combining exercise with a low-calorie diet can be especially effective for managing type 2 diabetes.

A study by Legrand & Heuzé (2007) examined how exercise can help reduce depression symptoms in people taking antidepressants. Over eight weeks, participants were divided into three groups: one group did low-frequency exercise, another did high-frequency exercise, and the third group combined high-frequency exercise with a group support setting. The results showed that those who exercised more frequently had greater reductions in their depression symptoms compared to the group that exercised less. This suggests that regular exercise can be a helpful addition to depression treatment to improve mood and to manage side effects like weight gain that can come with taking antidepressants.

The study suggests that exercise can be used as an adjunct therapy for depression and as a non-pharmacological intervention to prevent weight gain caused by some antidepressants such as Remeron.

Similarly, Effexor, a medication used to treat depression, anxiety, and panic disorders, has been found to cause sleep disturbances as a side effect. However, yoga has been found to alleviate insomnia. A study by Khalsa (2004) found that a simple daily yoga practice significantly improved sleep efficiency, total sleep time, and sleep onset latency in individuals with chronic insomnia. This suggests that yoga can be an effective non-pharmacological treatment for improving sleep quality.

Practices like mindfulness, meditation, and relaxation techniques can also help reduce insomnia. Establishing a calming bedtime routine with activities that promote relaxation can improve sleep quality for those experiencing sleep disturbances due to medication.

Integrating various therapeutic approaches, like psychotherapy, support groups, and self-help strategies, can address multiple aspects of mental health. By combining these approaches, you can take a more comprehensive and proactive stance in managing side effects and optimizing the benefits of your medication. A holistic approach that includes lifestyle changes, open communication, and personalized care contributes to a more effective and individualized mental health treatment plan.

Addressing Concerns: Busting Myths About Medication

There are a lot of questions and concerns floating around about medication and anxiety, and that's totally normal! After all, we're talking about something that directly impacts how we feel every day. But here's the thing: medication isn't something to be afraid of. In fact, it can be a game-changer for many people. So, let's dive in and clear up some of those common myths and concerns together.

First, anxiety and depression are really common. Millions of people deal with these issues, and while therapy, lifestyle changes, and things like exercise, meditation, and healthy eating can help, medication is often a key part of the treatment plan.

Now, let's bust the first myth: these medications aren't "happy pills." They don't magically make you feel good. What they actually do is help balance out the chemicals in your brain that can get out of balance when you're dealing with anxiety or depression. For instance, serotonin is a brain chemical that plays a big role in mood, sleep, and appetite. Medications like SSRIs work by making more serotonin available in your brain, which can help lift your mood and ease anxiety.

Another common worry is that if you start taking medication, you'll be stuck on it for life. This is not true! While some people might need long-term treatment, many others can eventually reduce or even stop their medication. This process, called tapering, is done gradually and under a doctor's supervision to make sure you don't have withdrawal symptoms or a return of your anxiety or depression.

For example, let's say someone has been on an antidepressant for six months and is feeling much better. Their doctor might suggest slowly lowering the dose over a few weeks or months. If all goes well, they might be able to stop taking the medication entirely.

And remember, medication isn't the only answer. Therapy, lifestyle changes, and holistic approaches can all play a big role in managing anxiety and depression. CBT helps people identify and change negative thought patterns that contribute to their feelings of anxiety or depression. Plus, regular exercise, a healthy diet, and good sleep can make a huge difference. Holistic practices like mindfulness, yoga, and even acupuncture can help reduce stress and promote relaxation.

In a nutshell, medication can be a really important part of treating anxiety and depression, but it's just one piece of the puzzle. By combining it with other approaches, you can effectively manage your symptoms and live a happier, healthier life.

5

NOURISHING THE MIND: THE ROLE OF NUTRITION IN MENTAL HEALTH

In this crucial chapter we dive into the powerful connection between what we eat and how we feel. It's not just about filling your stomach; it's about fueling your mind. Good nutrition is a game-changer when it comes to managing anxiety and depression. By understanding how your diet affects your mental health, you can make choices that boost your well-being.

As we explore the path to mental wellness, we'll uncover how nutrition shapes our psychological state. You'll learn about the science behind how certain nutrients, like omega-3 fatty acids, support brain function and mood regulation. Every meal becomes part of the bigger picture in maintaining a healthy, resilient mind.

In this chapter we'll highlight foods that can lift your mood and discuss the downsides of a diet lacking in essential nutrients, turning complex information into practical guidance. It's all about understanding how what you eat can directly influence your mental health. By the end of chapter 5, you'll have a clear understanding of how your dietary choices impact your mind. You'll be empowered to make decisions that nourish not just your body, but your mental well-being too. Your plate becomes a tool for building a stronger, more resilient you.

Understanding the Brain-Food Connection

Do you ever find yourself feeling a bit down or anxious for no obvious reason? It might have something to do with what's on your plate; or rather, what's missing from it. According to a study by the National Institutes of Health, certain nutrients like omega-3 fatty acids, B vitamins, and zinc are crucial for keeping our brains in top shape. When we don't get enough of these nutrients, it can actually make symptoms of depression and anxiety worse. But here's the good news: the right foods can give your brain the boost it needs to stay balanced and happy.

For example, foods rich in tryptophan, like turkey and eggs, can help your brain produce serotonin, that feel-good chemical that makes you happy. This chapter will help you understand these connections better so that the next time you're planning a meal, you can include nutrient-rich foods that nourish your body and keep your brain in a good mood.

The Gut-Brain Highway: Understanding the Gut-Brain Connection

Our bodies are complex, and none more so than the connection between our gut and our mental health, an area that's been receiving a lot of attention recently. Sometimes called our "second brain," the gut plays a huge role in how we feel mentally. The gut-brain axis is an amazing two-way communication system that links our digestive tract to our brain, and we're just starting to scratch the surface of how it all works. In the complex dance of our body's systems, the gut and brain are like best friends who are constantly chatting through a fascinating connection called the gut-brain axis. This special communication line, mainly run by the vagus nerve, links our digestive system directly to our brain, playing a big role in both our physical health and mental well-being.

The vagus nerve is the messenger between your gut and brain. It's a long nerve that acts like a two-way street, sending signals back and forth. This gut-brain axis isn't just about digestion; it's also about how you feel emotionally. Your gut is home to trillions of tiny microorganisms, called gut microbiota, that help regulate mood-related chemicals like neurotransmitters.

The gut and brain are in constant communication, and their conversations go far beyond digestion. They're actually discussing your mood and mental state too! Your gut microbiota play a big part in this, helping to produce and regulate the neurotransmitters that influence how you feel every day.

One of the gut-brain axis's key jobs is to help manage stress. In today's fast-paced world, stress is something we all deal with, and it can have a big impact on our mental health. The gut-brain axis helps fine-tune your body's response to stress, which is crucial for keeping anxiety and depression in check.

When it comes to anxiety and depression, understanding the gut-brain connection can be a real eye-opener. If the gut microbiota is out of balance, or if there's a glitch in the communication between the gut and brain, it can contribute to mood disorders. By keeping your gut healthy, you might be able to build a stronger foundation for better mental health.

Diving deeper into the gut-brain connection makes it clear that your digestive system isn't just about processing food. It's actively shaping your mental landscape too. That's why, in the upcoming chapters, we'll explore in greater detail how diet, lifestyle, and mindful choices can positively impact the gut-brain axis. I'll also offer practical tips along the way to help you nurture this powerful connection between your gut and mind.

The "Second Brain" Explained

Your gut is often called the "second brain" for good reason; it has its own network of millions of neurons, known as the enteric nervous system (ENS). This system can actually operate independently, managing digestion, absorption, and gut movement without constant input from your central nervous system.

Even though the enteric nervous system can do its own thing, it's still in constant communication with your central nervous system. This close connection means that what's happening in your gut can affect your brain, influencing your mood, emotions, and even cognitive function.

Understanding the enteric nervous system helps us see just how much wisdom is hidden in your gut. It's not just about digestion; it's about feeling, thinking, and living well. The term "second brain" really starts to make sense when you see how much power your gut has over your mental and emotional well-being.

Recent research also shows that your gut and brain are in sync with your gut microbiota—the tiny organisms living in your digestive system. They're constantly communicating, influencing each other, and even doing a little dance when it comes to your mental health.

A 2019 study by Peirce & Alviña found that stress can actually shake up your gut microbiota, which in turn can affect how you feel mentally. The researchers reviewed specific pathways through which the gut microbiome can influence the development of mental disorders such as depression and anxiety. They also discussed how stress-induced inflammation can harm brain function and affect mental health, highlighting the bidirectional communication between the gut and brain. This discovery highlights just how closely linked your gut health is to your overall mental state.

As we uncover more about the gut-brain connection, it's clear that these two aren't just working independently. They're a dynamic duo, constantly interacting, influencing each other, and keeping your mind and body in sync.

Keeping a healthy balance of gut bacteria is crucial for our mental well-being. When things get out of balance—something known as dysbiosis—it can increase the risk of anxiety and depression. Factors like diet, stress, and antibiotics can disrupt this balance, so it's definitely worth finding ways to support your gut health. After all, a happy gut can lead to a happier mind!

Food and Mood: the Impact of Diet on Mental Health

Let's talk about the powerful connection between what we eat and how we feel. Believe it or not, our food choices can have a big impact on our mental well-being, and understanding this link can help us make decisions that boost our mood and overall health. When it comes to our overall well-being, the importance of our diet cannot be overstated. Our gut health, in particular, is greatly affected by the foods we consume. While some foods, such as high-fiber options and fermented foods, promote a healthy gut, others can be incredibly harmful. A diet full of processed and sugary foods, for example, can hinder gut health and, by extension, our mental health.

A study by Bayes (2022) found that a Mediterranean diet packed with fruits, vegetables, lean proteins, and healthy fats can significantly improve depressive symptoms. Beyond the foods we eat, hydration also plays a crucial role in maintaining gut health. Ensuring proper water intake can keep the lining of our intestines healthy, supporting better nutrient absorption and overall gut health.

Imagine this: You've decided to overhaul your eating habits to boost your overall well-being. You start by ditching the fast food and sugary snacks that have been your go-to for quick meals. Instead, you switch to a Mediterranean diet, packed with fresh fruits, colorful vegetables, lean proteins like grilled chicken and fish, and healthy fats from nuts and olive oil.

As you make this change, you notice something surprising. You feel physically better, more energy, less bloating—and your mood starts to lift too! That lingering sense of sadness or anxiety starts to fade, and you begin to feel more positive and mentally sharp. This shift isn't just a coincidence; it's your gut and brain working together.

The high-fiber foods you're eating are feeding the good bacteria in your gut, and the fermented foods like yogurt and kimchi are adding even more beneficial microbes to the mix. Meanwhile, by cutting out processed foods and sugars, you're eliminating the bad actors that disrupt your gut's balance.

Foods That Boost Your Mood

Probiotics: the Gut's Friendly Bacteria. When it comes to keeping our gut in tip-top shape, probiotics are like the friendly superheroes we want on our side. These "good-guy" bacteria can have a big impact on our mental health, especially when it comes to managing anxiety and depression. Two of the standout strains are Lactobacillus and Bifidobacterium, which have shown real promise in helping with these issues. You can get your probiotic fix from a variety of delicious fermented foods like yogurt, kefir, sauerkraut, and kimchi, or even through dietary supplements. In fact, a recent study found that students who regularly ate probiotic-rich yogurt experienced lower levels of stress and anxiety.

Omega-3 Fatty Acids (Salmon, Chia Seeds). Did you know that foods rich in omega-3 fatty acids, like salmon and chia seeds, are great for your mental health? Harvard Medical School points out that these nutrients can help reduce symptoms of anxiety and depression. So adding more omega-3s to your diet could be a simple way to support your emotional well-being.

Complex Carbohydrates (Whole Grains). Whole grains, like oats and quinoa, are considered complex carbohydrates, and they do more than just fill you up. They help stabilize your blood sugar levels, which can prevent those pesky mood swings and keep your emotions more balanced.

Foods That Can Bring You Down

High-Sugar Foods. We all love a sweet treat now and then, but foods high in sugar can lead to a quick spike in energy followed by a "sugar crash." This crash can cause mood swings and leave you feeling tired and cranky, so it's a good idea to keep those sugary snacks in check.

Caffeine. A little caffeine can give you a nice boost, but too much can actually increase anxiety. The Mayo Clinic warns that if you're prone to anxiety, it's smart to monitor your caffeine intake to avoid unnecessary jitters.

Alcohol. While a drink might help you relax, the Mayo Clinic also notes that excessive alcohol can worsen depression. It's all about moderation; keeping your alcohol consumption in check can help protect your mood and mental health.

What we eat can play a huge role in how we feel. By choosing foods that support your mental well-being and being mindful of those that can negatively impact our mood, you can take an active role in nurturing your emotional health.

Meal Planning for Mental Health: Practical Tips to Incorporate Nutritious Foods

So now you know the important role nutrition plays in taking care of your mental health, you might be wondering how to start incorporating healthier foods. Here's how you can use meal planning to boost your mood and overall well-being:

1. Kickstart Your Day with a Balanced Breakfast

We've all heard that breakfast is the most important meal of the day, and there's a good reason for that! A balanced breakfast jump starts your metabolism and gives you the energy you need to tackle the day. By including protein, fiber, and healthy fats in your morning meal—like a veggie omelet with avocado—you help keep your blood sugar levels steady, which means fewer mood swings and less irritability.

2. Stay Hydrated

Did you know that even mild dehydration can mess with your mood and make it harder to concentrate? Water is essential for keeping everything in your body running smoothly, from transporting nutrients to flushing out waste. So keep a reusable water bottle handy and sip throughout the day to stay hydrated, mentally sharp, and feeling good.

3. Feed Your Brain with "Brain Foods"

Certain foods are like super fuel for your brain. Omega-3 fatty acids found in fish and walnuts are great for brain function and may help reduce inflammation. Antioxidant-rich foods like berries and leafy greens protect your brain from damage, while probiotics in yogurt and fermented foods support gut health, which is closely linked to mental health. Adding these "brain foods" to your meals can help keep your mind sharp and your mood balanced.

4. Watch Your Caffeine and Alcohol Intake

While a cup of coffee can help you stay alert, too much caffeine can lead to anxiety and mess with your sleep. Similarly, while a drink might help you relax, too much alcohol can actually worsen feelings of depression and anxiety. Keeping your caffeine and alcohol consumption in check can help you maintain a more stable mood and better mental health overall.

5. Start Small

Let's face it, overhauling your entire diet can feel overwhelming. The trick is to start small and make manageable changes. Try swapping refined grains for whole grains, or add a colorful serving of veggies to each meal.

These small tweaks can make a big difference over time, helping you build healthier habits that last.

6. Eat Mindfully

In today's busy world, eating often becomes just another task to check off. But mindful eating encourages us to slow down and really savor our food. By paying attention to each bite, avoiding distractions, and listening to our hunger cues, we can enjoy our meals more and even improve digestion and avoid overeating.

7. Get Professional and Personalized Nutrition Advice

With so many diet choices out there, it can be hard to know what's best for you. That's where a registered dietitian or nutritionist comes in. These pros can give you personalized advice tailored to your lifestyle and nutritional needs. Organizations like the Academy of Nutrition and Dietetics can help you find an expert who can assess your current diet and guide you toward healthier, more sustainable eating habits.

These meal planning tips are all about laying down a strong nutritional foundation for your mental well-being. By starting your day with a balanced breakfast, staying hydrated, incorporating brain-boosting foods, and being mindful of your caffeine and alcohol intake, you can help stabilize your blood sugar, nourish your brain, and reduce factors that contribute to anxiety and depression. And remember, these dietary strategies work best when combined with other healthy habits like regular exercise, good sleep, and stress management for a comprehensive approach to mental health, which we will look at in the coming chapters.

Before making any big changes to your diet or adding supplements, it's a good idea to check in with a healthcare provider or nutritionist. They can help you tailor your approach to fit your personal health needs, ensuring that you're making choices that are right for you.

In today's evolving approach to mental health, focusing on gut health is becoming a promising strategy. By making small, thoughtful changes to your lifestyle and diet, you can nurture your gut; and in turn your mental well-being, bringing more balance and resilience into your life.

Dietary Supplements: Do They Help?

Dietary supplements have become a hot topic when it comes to health and well-being. While it's always best to get the nutrients we need from a balanced diet, sometimes supplements can give us that extra boost—especially for our mental health. But not all supplements are the same, so it's important to do your homework before adding anything new to your routine. For some, the right supplements can make a big difference in mental clarity, mood, and overall well-being. Whether they support brain function, reduce inflammation, or provide essential vitamins and minerals, the right supplements can be a powerful tool in maintaining optimal mental health.

Omega-3 Supplements

Omega-3 fatty acids, particularly EPA and DHA, are superstars for brain health. They help reduce inflammation and are crucial for the structure and function of brain cells. Research published in the *Journal of Clinical Psychiatry* suggests that omega-3 supplements can effectively reduce symptoms of depression (Lespérance et al., 2011). This can be especially helpful for people who don't eat enough omega-3-rich foods like fatty fish. It's important to take omega-3 supplements in the right amounts and ideally under the guidance of a healthcare provider. Taking too much can lead to side effects or interactions with other medications.

Vitamin D Supplements

Vitamin D is key for many body functions, including keeping our mood in check. While we can get vitamin D from sunlight, supplements are beneficial for those who don't get enough sun exposure. Studies have linked low levels of vitamin D with depression. Supplementing with vitamin D can be particularly important for people who live in areas with little sunlight or during the winter months. Like with omega-3s, it's important to take vitamin D under a healthcare provider's supervision. Too much vitamin D can lead to toxicity, so regular monitoring is a good idea.

Personal Considerations

Not all supplements are created equal, and their effectiveness can depend on their form and quality. Choosing high-quality supplements with good bioavailability ensures your body can absorb them properly.

Before jumping into supplements, a healthcare provider might look at your diet to spot any nutritional gaps. Remember, a well-balanced diet should always be your primary source of essential nutrients.

In short, dietary supplements can be a helpful addition to support mental health, especially when addressing specific nutrient deficiencies. But it's important to approach them thoughtfully and with guidance from a healthcare professional to ensure they're both effective and safe. Always seek professional advice before adding new supplements to your routine.

While a balanced diet is crucial, and supplements are helpful, they are not cure-alls for mental health issues like anxiety or depression. True mental wellness comes from a combination of factors, including regular exercise, good sleep, stress management, and strong social connections. By integrating these elements into your life, you can create a more resilient and balanced mental state.

As you explore how to nourish your mind through diet, remember that this journey is uniquely yours. Use this chapter as a guide to help you make informed choices, take things at your own pace, and celebrate your progress. Embrace the changes, enjoy the process, and savor the benefits of a diet that fuels not just your body, but your mind and spirit too.

Your Voice Could Transform a Life

"Sometimes, the greatest gift you can give is a little hope." – Unknown

Understanding anxiety and depression is a journey, and sharing insights from this book can be a beacon of light for someone struggling in silence. That's why we have a heartfelt question for you:

Would you help someone you've never met, even if it didn't cost you anything?

If your answer is yes, we have a simple request – one that could profoundly impact someone else's life.

There are countless individuals out there, just like you, or perhaps like you were not long ago: seeking clarity, desperate for relief, and hoping for guidance to navigate the challenges of anxiety and depression.

You have the power to help them find this book.

How? Through a brief, honest review. It might seem small, but your review could be the very thing that inspires someone to take the next step toward understanding their struggles and finding hope.

Your review will:

- Help someone discover strategies to cope with anxiety and depression.

- Empower another individual to take control of their mental health journey.

- Encourage someone to embrace the possibility of healing.

- Be a ripple effect that changes lives.

It only takes 60 seconds to make a difference.

Here's how to leave your review on Amazon:

Scroll to the bottom of the book's page, click "Write a Review," and share your thoughts.

Or Scan Here!

P.S. Your support means the world to me, and your kindness in leaving a review allows this book to reach the people who need it most.

P.P.S. If you know someone who could benefit from *Understanding Anxiety and Depression,* consider sharing it with them. Your recommendation could make all the difference.

From the bottom of my heart, thank you. Your willingness to spread hope inspires us every day.

To Health and Healing,

Dr. A

6

Journey into Mindfulness: Your Secret Weapon Against Anxiety and Depression

The power of mindfulness and meditation is truly remarkable when it comes to managing anxiety and depression. In today's fast-paced world, it's all too easy to get caught up in the hustle and lose touch with ourselves. But taking just a few minutes to sit quietly and practice mindfulness can help us reconnect with our inner selves.

Mindfulness is all about being present in the moment and observing our thoughts without judgment. This simple practice can do wonders for easing anxiety and lifting the weight of depression. Meditation, on the other hand, helps us relax deeply, counteracting the harmful effects of stress on both our mind and body.

By making mindfulness and meditation part of your daily routine, you can tap into a powerful tool to combat anxiety and depression. It helps you stay grounded, calm, and in control, no matter what life throws your way.

Understanding Mindfulness: Why It Matters

Mindfulness, which has its roots in Buddhist traditions, is all about being fully present and engaged in the moment. It's about paying attention to your thoughts, feelings, and sensations without passing judgment on them. Over the years, mindfulness has become a big deal in Western psychology because it's been shown to reduce stress, improve focus, and boost emotional well-being.

Take, for example, a 2014 study by Johns Hopkins University, which found that mindfulness-based practices, like meditation, can help relieve psychological stresses such as anxiety, depression, and pain. Thanks to studies like this, mindfulness has become a go-to tool in many therapeutic settings.

One of the greatest aspects of mindfulness is how it helps you respond to your thoughts and feelings more intentionally. Instead of reacting impulsively or getting overwhelmed by emotions, mindfulness allows you to observe what's going on in your mind without judgment.

Remember Sarah, a busy professional who struggles with chronic stress? One morning, while working through a heavy task list, she gets a harsh email from her boss. Normally, she'd feel a wave of stress and irritation, maybe even fire off a snappy reply without thinking. But since she's started practicing mindfulness, she handles it differently.

When she reads the email, Sarah feels the stress and irritation bubbling up, but instead of reacting right away, she pauses. She takes a few deep breaths, giving herself a moment to really understand what she's feeling. She doesn't judge herself for being stressed; she just observes it. Then, with a clearer head, she decides to respond thoughtfully and constructively, rather than letting her emotions take the wheel.

This simple shift, from reacting impulsively to responding mindfully, shows how powerful mindfulness can be. It helps you manage stress, make better decisions, and keep your emotions in check. Mindfulness is a fantastic tool for navigating life's ups and downs. It gives you practical skills to handle stress, sharpen your focus, and lead a more balanced emotional life. As more and more people experience its benefits, mindfulness continues to shape the way we approach mental health and well-being. It is especially beneficial for those dealing with anxiety and depression, as meditation offers a sanctuary for self-reflection and a path toward greater emotional resilience.

Overcoming Obstacles: Making Mindfulness Work for You

Starting a mindfulness practice can be a daunting process. You may find yourself struggling to focus or feeling discouraged by intrusive thoughts. However, it's important to remember that obstacles are a normal part of the process. Mindfulness isn't about having a perfect practice but, rather, a consistent one. By persisting through these challenges, you'll learn to cultivate awareness and acceptance toward your own limitations.

Remember that mindfulness is a journey, not a destination, and every step counts toward improving your mental health. With dedication and patience, you can overcome the obstacles that arise and make mindfulness work for you. In the pursuit of mindfulness, common obstacles often surface, but with a flexible mindset and a gentle approach, these challenges can be transformed into opportunities for growth.

- **Time Constraints: Mindfulness on the Go.** One of the biggest hurdles people face is the belief that they just don't have time for mindfulness. But here's the great thing—mindfulness is super flexible. You don't need to carve out a big chunk of your day to practice it. You can sprinkle mindfulness into any moment, turning your daily routine into opportunities to be more present.

- **Wandering Minds: Embrace the Drift.** It's totally normal for your mind to wander during mindfulness exercises; everyone experiences this! The key is to gently guide your focus back to the present whenever you notice it drifting. It's a workout for your mindfulness muscle. Instead of getting frustrated, see these moments as part of the process and celebrate each time you bring your attention back.

- **Overcoming Skepticism: Keep an Open Mind.** Feeling skeptical about mindfulness? That's okay, especially if it's new to you. If you're not sure it's for you, try learning more about the science behind it or chat with someone who's found it helpful. Understanding why mindfulness works can help you approach it with an open mind.

Practical Steps to Incorporate Mindfulness into Your Life

Meditation isn't a one-size-fits-all practice. There are different paths you can take, each offering a unique approach to finding mental clarity and emotional balance.

- **Mindfulness Meditation:** This type encourages you to stay fully present in the moment, paying attention to your thoughts and feelings without getting caught up in them. It's about observing your mind without judgment.

- **Loving-Kindness Meditation:** This practice focuses on cultivating compassion and kindness toward yourself and others. It's a way to open your heart and gain deeper access to positive emotions.

- **Transcendental Meditation:** Aimed at reaching higher states of consciousness, this form of meditation involves repeating a mantra to help you transcend the noise of everyday thoughts and tap into a deeper state of awareness.

Each type of meditation offers its own journey, but they all lead to the same destination—a clearer mind and a more balanced emotional state.

The beauty of mindfulness is how effortlessly it can blend into your daily routines. It isn't about adding more to your plate; it's about shifting how you experience what's already there. For example, let's say you're brushing your teeth. Instead of letting your mind wander to your to-do list, try focusing on the sensation of the toothbrush against your teeth, the taste of the toothpaste, and the sound of the water. By paying attention to these details, you're practicing mindfulness.

Another everyday moment could be when you're having your morning coffee or tea. Instead of scrolling through your phone or mentally planning your day, take a moment to really savor the experience. Notice the warmth of the cup in your hands, the aroma rising from the drink, and the taste as you take that first sip. These small shifts in attention can turn routine activities into mindful practices.

You can also dedicate a few minutes each day to mindfulness meditation. Find a quiet space, focus on your breath or a specific sensation, and let thoughts come and go without judgment. Here is a creative visualization technique you can use when you are dedicating time to practicing:

- **Visualization:** Imagine your thoughts as leaves gently drifting down a serene stream. As you sit in quiet contemplation, envision each thought taking the form of a leaf, carried by the gentle current.

- **Acknowledgment:** As a leaf (thought) floats into your awareness, acknowledge it without judgment or analysis.

- **Release:** Instead of holding onto the leaf, let it continue its journey downstream. Watch it gracefully move away.

- **Detachment:** Feel a sense of detachment as each thought leaves your immediate focus. Recognize that thoughts come and go, much like the leaves on the stream.

- **Tranquility:** With each passing leaf, experience a growing sense of tranquility and inner calm.

This mental imagery reinforces the essence of mindfulness—observing thoughts without becoming entangled in them. It allows you to cultivate a peaceful detachment, promoting a more tranquil state of mind.

Mindfulness Apps: Your Pocket Guide

If you're new to mindfulness or need a little help getting started, apps like Calm or Headspace are fantastic resources. These apps offer guided mindfulness sessions that fit easily into your day, whether you have just a few minutes or a bit more time. For example, you might use a guided meditation from Headspace during your morning commute or a quick breathing exercise from Calm before bed. These tools make it easy to bring mindfulness into your daily life, no matter how busy you are.

Consistency is Key: Building the Habit

The power of mindfulness lies in regular practice. You don't need to spend hours meditating; just a few minutes each day can make a significant difference. For instance, you might start with a simple breathing exercise every morning. Doing this consistently can help you start your day with a clear and calm mind.

Over time you'll find that these small, consistent practices add up. You might notice that you're better able to handle stress, that you feel more grounded throughout the day, or that you're more attuned to your emotions. The key is to keep at it, even if it's just for a few minutes each day.

What's Next: Expanding Your Mindfulness Practice

As you get more comfortable with mindfulness, you can start exploring different techniques and incorporating them into various parts of your life. For example, as mindfulness becomes more of a subconscious habit, you might find you can practice mindfulness while also doing household chores like washing dishes or folding laundry.

Mindfulness can also be a part of your social interactions. When you're having a conversation with someone, practice being fully present. Listen attentively without thinking about what you're going to say next. Notice the other person's expressions and tone of voice. This improves your communication and strengthens your connections with others.

In essence, mindfulness is about being present and fully engaged in the moments that make up your life. By incorporating these small practices into your day, you can cultivate a greater sense of peace, clarity, and emotional balance. Over time, mindfulness can become second nature; a way of life that enhances your overall well-being.

So the next time you're brushing your teeth, sipping your coffee, or walking to work, remember that these are all opportunities to practice mindfulness. With a little intention and consistency, you can turn these everyday moments into powerful practices that support your mental and emotional health.

Mindfulness for Anxiety: a Calm Port in the Storm

So now we've looked at how mindfulness is all about staying fully present and aware of what's happening right now, without getting caught up in judgment about the future or the past, let's focus on how mindfulness helps anxiety. It can be a powerful tool for managing anxiety by helping you develop a healthier relationship with your thoughts and emotions. Here's how it works:

Breaking the Cycle of Negative Thoughts

Anxiety often comes from getting stuck in a loop of negative thoughts—worrying about the future, fearing the worst, or dwelling on past mistakes. Mindfulness helps you become aware of these thoughts without getting caught up in them. Instead of spiraling into anxiety, you learn to observe your thoughts as they come and go, which can help break the cycle and reduce the intensity of your anxiety.

For example, let's say you've got a big presentation coming up at work, and you start thinking, "I'm going to mess up" or "Everyone's going to judge me." Instead of spiraling into those negative thoughts, mindfulness teaches you to notice them without getting sucked in. You might think, "Okay, I'm feeling nervous, but that doesn't mean I'll fail." This way, you acknowledge the thoughts but don't let them run the show.

Grounding Yourself in the Present

Anxiety often pulls you out of the present moment, making you worry about events that haven't happened yet or things that are out of your control. Mindfulness brings your attention back to the here and now. By focusing on your breath, bodily sensations, or your surroundings, you can ground yourself in the present moment, which helps to calm your mind and reduce anxiety.

Imagine you're having a hectic day, and stress is piling up. Take a quick mindfulness break—close your eyes, breathe deeply, and focus on the sensation of your breath coming in and out. Just a few moments of this can help you hit the reset button and find a little peace amidst the chaos.

Creating a Pause Before Reacting

When you're anxious, it's easy to react impulsively to your emotions. Mindfulness creates a space between your thoughts and your reactions, allowing you to respond to situations more calmly and thoughtfully. This can help prevent anxiety from escalating and give you more control over how you handle stressful situations.

For example, if you're feeling stressed about an upcoming job interview, mindfulness helps you pull your focus back to the here and now. Instead of obsessing over what might happen, try grounding yourself by feeling your feet on the floor or noticing the texture of something in your hand. This helps you stay present rather than getting lost in future "what-ifs."

Building Emotional Resilience

Mindfulness helps you develop a non-judgmental awareness of your emotions, including anxiety. Instead of trying to push anxiety away or feeling bad about feeling anxious, mindfulness teaches you to accept it as part of your experience. This acceptance can reduce the power anxiety has over you and build emotional resilience, making it easier to cope with anxiety when it arises.

When you're in the middle of a panic attack, it can feel overwhelming. Mindfulness techniques like focused breathing can be a lifesaver. Try diaphragmatic breathing—taking slow, deep breaths from your belly. This calms your nervous system and shifts your focus away from the intense anxiety, helping you regain control.

Reducing Physical Symptoms of Anxiety

Anxiety often comes with physical symptoms like a racing heart, shallow breathing, or muscle tension. Mindfulness practices, such as deep breathing exercises or progressive muscle relaxation, can help soothe these physical symptoms. By calming your body, you also help calm your mind, which can significantly reduce anxiety levels.

Suppose you're feeling anxious before a social event. Instead of beating yourself up for being nervous, mindfulness encourages you to be kind to yourself. You might think, "It's okay to feel this way; it's just my body's way of preparing." Then, you can go into the event without letting those anxious feelings dictate your actions.

Improving Self-Awareness

Mindfulness increases your awareness of what triggers your anxiety and how it manifests in your body and mind. With this heightened self-awareness, you can start to recognize early signs of anxiety and take steps to manage it before it becomes overwhelming. If you're anxious about a looming deadline, mindfulness reminds you that this feeling isn't permanent. By recognizing that emotions are like waves in how they rise and fall, you can approach your work with a calmer mindset, knowing that the anxiety will pass.

Encouraging Self-Compassion

Mindfulness encourages a kind and compassionate attitude toward yourself. When you're anxious, it's easy to be hard on yourself or feel frustrated that you're struggling. Mindfulness teaches you to treat yourself with the same kindness and understanding you would offer a friend, which can help ease the burden of anxiety.

Mindfulness for Depression: Shedding Light on the Shadows

Depression can feel like a heavy shadow that follows you everywhere, casting a gloom over even the brightest moments. It's a condition that can deeply affect how you think, feel, and interact with the world. But mindfulness offers a way to shed light on those shadows, helping to manage depression by changing how you relate to your thoughts and emotions.

When you're depressed, it's easy to get trapped in a cycle of negative thinking. You might find yourself constantly ruminating on past mistakes or worrying about the future. Mindfulness helps by teaching you to observe these thoughts without getting tangled up in them.

Take Abigail, a thirty-five-year-old who recently lost her job. She's been plagued by thoughts like, "I'm worthless" or "I'll never find another job." Through mindfulness, Abigail learns to notice these thoughts as they arise, but instead of letting them spiral out of control, she observes them with curiosity. Instead, she thinks, "There's that thought again," without immediately accepting it as the truth. Over time, she realizes that these thoughts are just that—thoughts—and not an accurate reflection of who she is or her future.

Finding Success with Mindfulness-Based Cognitive Therapy (MBCT)

Mindfulness-based cognitive therapy (MBCT) is a structured program that combines the principles of cognitive therapy with mindfulness practices. It's designed to help people who have experienced repeated bouts of depression by preventing the downward spiral into another episode.

Let's look at James, a forty-year-old who has faced recurring depression. He decides to try MBCT after experiencing side effects from antidepressants. Through the program, James learns to recognize the early warning signs of depression, such as feelings of hopelessness or a loss of interest in activities. Instead of letting these feelings take over, he uses mindfulness techniques to step back and view his thoughts objectively. One such technique is to engage in a body scan meditation, where he slowly focuses on different parts of his body, noticing any tension or discomfort without judgment. This helps him stay grounded and prevents his thoughts from snowballing into a full-blown depressive episode. The success of MBCT is well-documented, with studies like the 2015 research by Kuyken et al. that was published in *The Lancet* showing that it can be as effective as antidepressants in preventing relapse.

Boosting Positive Emotions with Loving-Kindness Meditation

Depression often brings a sense of numbness or a lack of positive emotions. Loving-kindness meditation is a mindfulness practice that focuses on developing feelings of compassion and love, both for yourself and others.

Justina, a twenty-eight-year-old who struggles with self-loathing, finds it difficult to experience joy in her daily life. She begins practicing loving-kindness meditation, where she silently repeats phrases like, "May I be happy, may I be healthy, may I live with ease." Over time she extends these wishes to others, starting with loved ones and gradually including even those she has conflicts with. This practice helps Justina cultivate a sense of warmth and connection, countering the isolation and negativity that often accompany depression. She begins to notice small moments of happiness and appreciation in her daily life, which contributes to an overall shift in her emotional state.

Changing the Relationship with Negative Feelings

Depression is often accompanied by a flood of negative emotions—sadness, guilt, anger, to name a few—that can feel overwhelming. Mindfulness encourages a change in relationship with these feelings by observing them without trying to push them away.

Alex, the forty-five-year-old banking executive we looked at earlier who is struggling at work, feels inadequate because he's struggling to find success in the workplace. His depression is fueled by these feelings of failure. Through mindfulness, Alex learns to acknowledge his emotions without immediately reacting to them. He notices the tightness in his chest when he feels anxious or the heaviness in his limbs when he's sad. Instead of trying to suppress these feelings, he accepts them as a natural part of his experience. This acceptance doesn't mean giving in to the feelings; it means recognizing them without letting them control his actions. As Alex practices this non-judgmental awareness, he begins to see that these feelings, while intense, are not permanent and do not define him. One of the challenges of depression is the belief that your current emotional state will last forever. Mindfulness helps you see that emotions, like all experiences, are temporary.

For example, Maria, a thirty-year-old artist, is frustrated by a creative block that's fueling her depression. She's worried that she'll never produce good work again. Through mindfulness, Maria starts to observe her emotions without getting wrapped up in them. One of the phrases she tells herself is, "I'm feeling stuck right now, but this will pass." By recognizing that her frustration is temporary, she's able to approach her creative work with more patience and less self-criticism. This perspective helps her ride out the low points, knowing that they don't define her or her abilities as an artist.

Reflecting Mindfully for Balanced Well-Being

However, mindfulness isn't just about managing negative emotions; it's also about cultivating a balanced, reflective approach to life.

To illustrate, let's look at Tom, a fifty-year-old executive, who feels overwhelmed by the chronic stress of his job, which has led to depression. He decides to integrate mindfulness into his daily routine. Tom starts with simple practices, like taking a few deep breaths before important meetings or spending a few minutes in the evening reflecting on his day. These moments of mindfulness help him become more aware of how his thoughts and emotions are connected. As a result of this, he notices that his stress peaks when he skips lunch to power through work. With this awareness, Tom makes small changes to his routine, taking regular breaks and eating meals mindfully. These adjustments help him manage his stress better, leading to a more balanced and fulfilling life.

Mindfulness offers a powerful way to manage depression by changing how you relate to your thoughts and emotions. It's not about eliminating negative feelings or trying to be happy all the time. Instead, it's about developing a more compassionate, accepting relationship with your experiences. By practicing mindfulness, you can shed light on the shadows of depression, helping you navigate the ups and downs of life with greater resilience and ease. Whether it's through breaking free from negative thought patterns, learning to accept emotions without judgment, or recognizing the temporary nature of feelings, mindfulness provides practical tools for living a more balanced and emotionally healthy life.

7

A Breath of Fresh Air: Exploring Aromatherapy for Anxiety and Depression

In the hustle and bustle of modern life, the search for tranquility often leads us down various avenues. In this quest the age-old practice of aromatherapy emerges as a breath of fresh air, a therapeutic journey entwined with the essence of nature. With stress and anxiety becoming an increasingly common part of our daily lives, it's no wonder that more and more people are looking toward unconventional approaches to manage their mental health.

Aromatherapy, the practice of using essential oils extracted from plants and other natural sources, has become a go-to for many individuals seeking a more natural and holistic approach to managing anxiety and depression. The fragrant properties of essential oils have long been known to possess a soothing and calming effect on the mind and body, making them an incredibly accessible tool for anyone seeking relief. In this chapter we explore the world of aromatherapy and how it can be used to help alleviate the symptoms of anxiety and depression.

The Scent-sational Basics of Aromatherapy

There's something magical about a great smell; it can whisk you back to a favorite memory, stir up powerful emotions, or even give your body a boost. That's the idea behind aromatherapy. The secret? The scent receptors in our noses send signals straight to the brain's limbic system, which is the part of the brain that handles emotions. By tapping into this, aromatherapy can help calm a busy mind, re-energize a tired body, or just make a space feel more welcoming. Whether you're a seasoned pro or just dipping your toes into the world of aromatherapy, it's hard to deny the "scent-sational" benefits once you've experienced them.

Picking the Perfect Essential Oil

Choosing the right essential oil is key to getting the most out of aromatherapy, and it's not just about the scent! With so many oils out there, it's important to go for 100 percent pure options that don't have any synthetic additives. The quality of an essential oil can be influenced by factors such as where the plant was grown, how it was harvested, and the methods used to extract the oil. But before you dive in, remember that not all oils are skin-friendly. Some can cause irritation or even allergic reactions. It's a good idea to do a patch test first and always dilute the essential oil with a carrier oil like coconut or jojoba before applying it to your skin. This way, you can enjoy the benefits without any unwanted side effects.

By taking the time to pick high-quality oils and using them safely, you can fully enjoy the perks of aromatherapy. Whether you're looking to relax, energize, or simply add a little extra joy to your day, essential oils can be a powerful tool in your wellness toolkit. So go ahead, explore the world of aromatherapy and let your nose lead the way to better well-being!

The Aroma Arsenal: Essential Oils for Anxiety and Depression

Among the many options out there, a few essential oils stand out for their ability to ease anxiety and lift your mood. Let's dive into some of the best essential oils you can add to your "aroma arsenal."

Lavender: the Go-To for Relaxation and Sleep

Lavender is like the superstar of essential oils when it comes to relaxation. This sweet-smelling oil is renowned for its calming effects. And it's not just hype; there's solid science behind it. A study by Kasper et al. (2010) found that lavender oil is effective in managing anxiety and insomnia. When you inhale lavender, apply it to your skin, or even add a few drops to your bath, it works its magic by calming your nervous system. And the benefits don't stop there—lavender can also improve your sleep quality, boost concentration, and lift your mood. So the next time you're feeling stressed or having trouble sleeping, reach for some lavender oil and let it work its calming wonders.

Chamomile: the Calming Classic

If you're searching for a natural way to reduce anxiety, chamomile might just be your new best friend. This gentle, soothing plant is famous for its use in teas, but its calming properties go beyond just a warm beverage. Chamomile has been scientifically shown to help with anxiety too. A study published in *Phytomedicine* found that chamomile capsules provided a mild benefit in treating generalized anxiety disorder (Amsterdam et al., 2009). It's also been praised for promoting better sleep and reducing stress, according to a review in the *Asian Pacific Journal of Tropical Biomedicine*. So if you're feeling frazzled, why not brew yourself a cup of chamomile tea or use chamomile oil? It's a simple, natural way to find your inner calm.

Ylang-Ylang: the Mood Booster

Looking for a way to uplift your spirits and ease stress naturally? Enter ylang-ylang, an exotic flower with a sweet, floral aroma that's as soothing as it is fragrant. Ylang-ylang is known for its ability to promote feelings of comfort and joy. Research published in the *Complementary Therapies in Clinical Practice* journal shows that inhaling ylang-ylang oil can significantly reduce stress levels. And it gets even better, another study in *Phytotherapy Research* found that when ylang-ylang is used in a blend with lavender and bergamot, it can greatly reduce psychological stress and lower cortisol levels, the hormone associated with stress. So the next time you're feeling anxious or overwhelmed, try adding ylang-ylang oil to your routine and let its calming scent help you relax.

Start with a Diffuser: Style Meets Serenity

If you're new to aromatherapy, investing in an essential oil diffuser is a great way to get started. These nifty gadgets break down essential oils into tiny molecules and spread their aroma throughout your space. They make your home smell amazing, and they can also help you unwind after a long day. And if you're worried about clashing with your decor, no need—brands like Vitruvi offer diffusers that are as stylish as they are functional. Just add a few drops of your favorite oil, kick back, and breathe easy knowing you're doing something good for both your body and mind. However, you don't need a diffuser to enjoy the benefits of essential oils. Here are some other fun and easy ways to incorporate them into your life:

Inhalation Methods

- **Steam Inhalation:** Got a cold or just need to clear your head? Add a few drops of essential oil to a bowl of hot water. Lean over it with a towel draped over your head, and breathe in the steam.

- **Direct Inhalation:** Sometimes, simple is best. Open the bottle and inhale directly, or place a few drops on a washcloth and hold it close to your nose for an instant pick-me-up.

Topical Application

- **Dilution is Key:** If you want to apply essential oils directly to your skin, always mix them with a carrier oil like coconut, almond, or jojoba oil to avoid irritation.

- **Massage:** Combine your chosen essential oil with a carrier oil for a relaxing massage. This way, you enjoy the scent and get the soothing physical benefits of a massage.

DIY Room Spray

- **Freshen Up:** Mix water with a few drops of essential oil in a spray bottle, and voilà! You've got yourself a natural air freshener. Perfect for spritzing around the house or even on your sheets before bedtime.

Take Aromatherapy On-the-Go

Why limit the goodness of essential oils to your home? Here are some ways to keep those calming scents with you all day:

- **Aromatherapy Jewelry:** Beyond necklaces and bracelets, you can find diffuser rings and earrings that let you carry your favorite scents with you. Stylish and soothing!

- **Car Diffusers:** Keep your car smelling fresh and calming by using a portable diffuser or simply adding a few drops of oil to a cotton ball and placing it in the air vent.

- **Scented Clay Discs:** These handy little discs absorb essential oils and slowly release the scent. Pop one in your bag, drawer, or car for a subtle, long-lasting fragrance.

Get Creative

Feeling crafty? Here are a few DIY ideas to get even more out of your essential oils:

- **DIY Reed Diffusers:** Mix essential oils with a carrier oil, place reed sticks in the jar, and let the scent naturally diffuse throughout the room.

- **Candle Infusion:** Before lighting an unscented candle, add a few drops of essential oil to the wax. As the candle burns, it will fill the room with your chosen aroma.

Essential oils are powerful, so it's important to use them safely. Always do a little research on each oil's properties, especially if you're planning to apply them to your skin. A patch test and proper dilution are key to avoiding any unwanted reactions.

With these tips and tricks, you can easily make aromatherapy a natural part of your daily routine. Whether you're looking to relax, energize, or just enjoy a lovely scent, there's an essential oil—and a method—that's perfect for you. So go ahead, breathe deeply and let the magic of aromatherapy enhance your everyday life!

A Word of Caution: Safety and Aromatherapy

It's important to note that while essential oils have benefits, they can also be harmful if not used properly. In fact, some essential oils can even be toxic if ingested or applied incorrectly. It's important to take the necessary precautions to ensure you are safely using aromatherapy. This includes doing research on the proper usage of essential oils, using high-quality products, and following instructions carefully. By practicing caution and taking these steps, you can safely enjoy the benefits of aromatherapy without risking harm to yourselves or others.

Special consideration should be paid to the following groups when using aromatherapy around them:

- **Pregnant women and Nursing Mothers.** Caution should be exercised around pregnant women and nursing mothers when using essential oils, as some oils may have effects on hormone levels or may not be suitable during pregnancy. Consult with a healthcare professional before using essential oils to find out which ones are safe for use.

- **Children and Pets.** Essential oils should be used with caution around children and pets. Some oils can be toxic to them, and certain diffusion methods might not be suitable. Always keep oils out of reach of children.

- **Medical Conditions.** Individuals with certain medical conditions, such as asthma or epilepsy, should consult with a healthcare provider before using essential oils, as some oils may trigger reactions.

- **Respiratory Sensitivity.** People with respiratory issues or sensitivities should be cautious with strong essential oils, especially those with high menthol content.

It's also a good idea to consider these factors when using essential oils:

- **Quality Matters.** Ensure that you are using high-quality, pure essential oils. Lower-quality oils may contain additives that can cause adverse reactions.

- **Use in Enclosed Spaces.** When using essential oils in enclosed spaces, ensure proper ventilation to prevent the concentration of vapors, which can be overwhelming.

- **Storage.** Store essential oils in dark glass bottles, away from direct sunlight, heat, and moisture. This helps preserve their quality over time.

- **Adherence to Guidelines.** Follow recommended dilution ratios when applying essential oils to the skin. Different oils have different dilution guidelines, and adherence to these ratios helps prevent skin irritation.

- **Mindful Diffusion.** Be mindful of the duration and intensity of diffusion. Prolonged exposure to concentrated essential oil vapors can lead to discomfort or irritation.

By prioritizing safety and being aware of individual sensitivities, you can maximize the benefits of aromatherapy while minimizing potential risks. If in doubt, seeking advice from a qualified healthcare professional is always a prudent step, especially for those with pre-existing health conditions or those taking prescribed medications.

8

Unwind Your Mind: Exploring Relaxation Techniques for Anxiety and Depression

As we discussed in chapter 1, the stresses of daily life can often leave us feeling overwhelmed, anxious, and depressed. Luckily, there are ways to combat these negative emotions and improve our mental wellbeing. By practicing relaxation techniques, we can unwind our minds and find a sense of calm even in the midst of chaos. These techniques can include deep breathing exercises, progressive muscle relaxation, guided imagery, and more. Whether it's taking a few deep breaths before a big meeting or dedicating some time each day to practicing these techniques, incorporating relaxation into our lives can make a world of difference in managing anxiety and depression.

These techniques work to reduce stress levels, and they promote a sense of mindfulness and self-awareness. This chapter will give you practical strategies to help you unwind your mind so you can see the positive impact it can have on your mental health.

Deep Breathing: More than Just Inhale and Exhale

As humans, we often take our breath for granted. It's always there, constantly working to keep us alive without us even realizing it. But the power of our breath goes beyond just keeping us alive; it can also be harnessed to keep us calm and centered. Deep breathing is one technique that can help us achieve a state of relaxation in times of stress. By taking slow, conscious breaths, we can bring more oxygen into our bodies and lower our heart rate, which leads to a sense of calm and clarity.

Incorporating deep breathing exercises into your daily routine can have a profound impact on your mental and physical well-being, helping to calm your mind and release tension from your body. One easy way to get started with deep breathing is to take a few moments each day to sit or lay down somewhere comfortable, then inhale deeply through your nose for a count of four before exhaling slowly through your mouth for another four counts. Repeat this process for five to ten cycles, allowing yourself to fully exhale each time. With a little practice, you'll find yourself feeling more grounded and centered in no time!

By intentionally taking deep breaths, you stimulate the body's relaxation response. This can lead to a decreased heart rate, lower blood pressure, and an overall sense of well-being. The beauty of deep breathing is that it can be practiced anywhere and at any time, making it a valuable tool for anyone looking to reduce stress in their lives. Whether you're a busy executive, a harried parent, or a student navigating the pressures of academia, taking a few moments to practice deep breathing can help you feel more centered and grounded throughout your day.

So why not try it out during your next lunch break at work? It may just be the calming, rejuvenating break your body and mind need.

The 4-7-8 breathing technique has been gaining popularity in recent years for its reported effectiveness. By inhaling for four seconds, holding for seven, and exhaling for eight, this technique can help slow down the heart rate and improve oxygen flow to the brain.

Understanding the 4-7-8 Method

The 4-7-8 deep breathing technique is like a magic trick for your mind and body, designed to help you relax by controlling your breath. Each step—inhaling, holding, and exhaling—has a special role in activating your body's natural relaxation response.

- **Inhale (four seconds):** Start by taking a slow, deep breath in through your nose for a count of four seconds. Imagine filling your lungs completely, letting your belly rise as you breathe in.

- **Hold (seven seconds):** After inhaling, hold your breath for seven seconds. This pause gives your body a chance to fully absorb the oxygen and allows you to settle into a moment of stillness.

- **Exhale (eight seconds):** Breathe out slowly through pursed lips for a count of eight seconds. Focus on releasing all the air from your lungs, letting go of any tension as you exhale.

How to Practice the 4-7-8 Method

1. **Find Your Calm Spot.** Start by finding a quiet, comfortable place where you won't be disturbed. Sit or lie down in a relaxed position.

2. **Get Your Posture Right.** If you're sitting, keep your back straight and your shoulders relaxed. If you're lying down, ensure your spine is aligned. Place one hand on your abdomen to feel the rise and fall of your breath.

3. **Start with the Inhale.** Inhale gently through your nose for four seconds. Focus on the air filling your lungs and your belly expanding with the breath.

4. **Hold It In.** After you've inhaled, hold your breath for seven seconds. Embrace the pause, and let yourself be fully present in the moment.

5. **Slowly Exhale.** Exhale through pursed lips for eight seconds, letting all the air out and feeling your body relax with each breath out.

6. **Repeat the Cycle.** Go through this 4-7-8 cycle at least three times to start. As you get more comfortable, you can increase the number of cycles.

Tips for Success

- **Practice Regularly.** Make the 4-7-8 method a part of your daily routine so it becomes second nature.

- **Quality over Quantity.** Focus on the quality of each breath rather than rushing through the counts. Slow and steady wins the race here.

- **Find Your Moment.** Try this technique at different times of the day, whether it's during a stressful moment, before bed, or whenever you need a quick calm-down.

The 4-7-8 method is a relaxation hack you can use anytime, anywhere. With consistent practice, it can become your go-to tool for finding calm, easing anxiety, and promoting overall well-being. So the next time you feel stressed or just need a moment to unwind, give the 4-7-8 a try and breathe your way to a better state of mind!

Progressive Muscle Relaxation: Tense to Relax

If you're searching for a way to truly relax and let go of the day's stress, progressive muscle relaxation (PMR) might just become your new best friend.

PMR is a technique that involves systematically tensing and then relaxing different muscle groups to promote physical and mental relaxation. Developed by Edmund Jacobson in the early twentieth century, PMR is widely used for stress management and improving overall well-being.

Think of PMR as a gentle dance of tensing and releasing, moving through your body like a soothing wave. As you tense each muscle group, you become more aware of how stress feels in your body. Then, when you release that tension, you experience the sweet relief of letting go. This process eases physical tension and helps calm your mind, creating a bridge from anxiety to relaxation. By consciously tensing and relaxing your muscles, you become more attuned to the difference between stress and relaxation. This awareness is key to guiding your mind away from anxiety and into a state of peace.

For those dealing with anxiety or depression, falling asleep can be a challenge. But PMR can act like a soothing lullaby, helping you drift off into a peaceful slumber. Picture yourself lying in bed, starting with your toes and gradually working your way up to your head. As you move from one muscle group to the next, tensing and then releasing, you'll feel the stress of the day melt away, leaving you ready for a restful night.

How to Get Started with PMR

Getting started with PMR is simple, but the benefits can be profound. Let's break it down step by step so you can make the most of this relaxation technique and incorporate it into your daily routine.

Find Your Sanctuary

First things first, create your relaxation space. You want to find a quiet, cozy spot where you can fully relax without interruptions. This could be your bed, a comfortable chair, or even a yoga mat on the floor. The key is to make sure you're comfortable and that your environment is conducive to relaxation.

- **Create a Relaxing Atmosphere.** Dim the lights, play some soft music, or light a scented candle. This helps set the mood for relaxation.

- **Dress Comfortably.** Wear loose, comfortable clothing that doesn't restrict your movement or breathing.

- **Disconnect.** Turn off any distractions, like your phone or TV, to fully immerse yourself in the experience.

Begin Your Toe-to-Head Journey

Now let's get into the practice itself. PMR works by systematically tensing and then relaxing each muscle group in your body. You'll start from your toes and work your way up to your head, spending about five to ten seconds on each muscle group.

- **Start with Your Toes.** Begin by focusing on your toes. Tense them as tightly as you can for about five seconds. Feel the tension build up. Then, release and let your toes relax completely. Notice the contrast between the tension and relaxation.

- **Move Up Your Body.** After your toes, move on to your feet. Tense them, hold for a few seconds, and then release. Continue this process with your calves, thighs, buttocks, abdomen, chest, arms, hands, shoulders, neck, and finally, your face.

- **Be Gentle.** Don't overdo the tensing. You want to feel the muscles engage, but not to the point of discomfort. The goal is to heighten your awareness of each muscle group.

Embrace the Mindful Meltdown

As you move through each muscle group, stay mindful of the sensations in your body. This is where the magic of PMR happens—by focusing on how your body feels as you tense and release, you're not just relaxing physically, but also calming your mind.

- **Stay Present.** Focus on each muscle group as you work through the sequence. If your mind starts to wander, gently bring it back to the sensations in your body.

- **Feel the Release.** Notice how each part of your body feels after you release the tension. Pay attention to the feeling of relaxation spreading through your body.

- **Breathe Deeply.** Coordinate your breathing with the tensing and relaxing. Inhale as you tense the muscles and exhale as you release. This helps deepen the relaxation effect.

Bask in Bedtime Bliss

Once you've worked through your entire body, take a few moments to simply be. This is your time to enjoy the calm and tranquility you've created.

- **Lie Still.** After completing the toe-to-head journey, lie quietly for a few minutes. Let your body sink into your bed or chair, and relish the sensation of total relaxation.

- **Reflect on the Calm.** Take note of how different your body feels compared to when you started. This reflection reinforces the relaxation response and helps train your mind to recognize the benefits of PMR.

- **Drift into Sleep.** If you're practicing PMR at bedtime, let this calmness carry you into a restful sleep. Allow the relaxation to guide you naturally into slumber.

Tips for Success

- **Consistency is Key.** Try to practice PMR daily, especially before bed. The more consistent you are, the more natural and effective the technique becomes.

- **Adapt to Your Needs.** If you're short on time, you can focus on just a few muscle groups. Alternatively, if you have more time, you can spend longer on each part of your body.

- **Combine with Other Relaxation Techniques.** PMR works well alongside other relaxation practices, such as deep breathing, meditation, or listening to calming music.

By following these steps, you can make progressive muscle relaxation a powerful tool in your stress-relief arsenal. It's a simple yet effective way to unwind, de-stress, and set yourself up for a peaceful night's sleep. So find your sanctuary, start your toe-to-head journey, and let the relaxation begin!

Making PMR a Nightly Ritual

Incorporating PMR into your nightly routine can signal to your body that it's time to unwind. You can even pair it with soothing music or nature sounds to enhance the experience. Be patient with yourself; like any new habit, the more you practice PMR, the easier it will be to slip into relaxation mode and enjoy a restful night.

Progressive muscle relaxation isn't just a technique; it's an invitation to reclaim your nights, let go of tension, and embrace the tranquility that's waiting for you. Make your bedtime a sanctuary of peace, and let PMR guide you to a place of deep, restorative sleep.

Visualization: a Mental Escape

In our fast-paced, always-on world, finding a moment of peace can feel like a luxury. But what if you could escape to a tranquil place anytime you wanted, even if just for a few minutes? Visualization, a technique that involves creating a mental image of a calming scene, offers just that—a mental vacation that's only a few deep breaths away.

The Power of Your Imagination

By harnessing the power of your imagination, you can transport yourself to a place where stress doesn't exist. Picture yourself on a serene beach, with waves gently lapping at the shore, the warmth of the sun on your skin, and the scent of salty sea air filling your lungs. Whether it's a cozy cabin in the woods or a tropical paradise, you can create your own mental oasis tailored to what relaxes you most.

Also known as guided imagery, visualization is a widely practiced technique for relaxation and stress reduction. It's simple to get started, and you don't need any special skills, just a willingness to let your mind wander to peaceful places. Apps like Insight Timer and Smiling Mind offer a range of guided visualization exercises, making it easy for beginners to dive in.

How to Practice Visualization

Let's walk through a simple visualization exercise that combines progressive muscle relaxation (PMR) with guided imagery for a truly immersive experience:

1. **Set the Scene:**

    - Find a quiet, comfortable spot where you won't be disturbed. This could be your bed, a comfy chair, or even a yoga mat.

    - Use an app like Insight Timer to select a guided imagery session that resonates with you.

2. **Start with PMR:**

    - Begin by tensing and then relaxing each muscle group, starting from your toes and working your way up to your head. As you release the tension, visualize yourself stepping into a serene beach setting.

    - Imagine the warmth of the sun, the softness of the sand beneath your feet, and the rhythmic sound of waves gently crashing.

3. **Engage Your Senses:**

    - Make the visualization as vivid as possible. Feel the sun's warmth, hear the distant call of seagulls, and smell the salty ocean breeze. The more you engage your senses, the more immersive and effective the experience will be.

4. **Sync Visualization with Relaxation:**

    - As you move through each muscle group, deepen the visualization. For example, as you release tension in your shoulders, picture the waves washing away any stress, leaving you calm and refreshed.

5. **Enjoy the Calm:**

    ◦ After you've completed the PMR session, take a few moments to simply enjoy the tranquility. Let your mind bask in the peaceful scene you've created, allowing the calm to carry you into a restful state.

Enhancing Your Visualization Practice

To get the most out of visualization, try these tips:

- **Experiment with Different Scenes:** Not everyone finds the beach relaxing, so feel free to explore other scenes like a quiet forest, a blooming meadow, or a tranquil mountain retreat.

- **Make It a Habit:** Consistency is key. Incorporate guided imagery into your daily routine, especially before bed, to enhance your relaxation experience.

- **Explore Different Apps:** Apps like Insight Timer and Smiling Mind offer a variety of guided visualizations. Try different sessions to find what works best for you.

Combining progressive muscle relaxation with guided imagery transforms your relaxation routine into a powerful mental and physical escape. It becomes more than just about releasing physical tension;, it also creates a sanctuary in your mind where you can retreat whenever you need a break from the chaos of life.

So the next time stress starts to creep in, remember that a peaceful escape is just a few deep breaths away. Let visualization guide you to your own personal oasis, where calm and tranquility await.

Autogenic Training: Harnessing the Power of Self-Suggestion

Imagine a technique that allows you to tap into your mind's ability to create calm and relaxation, all through the power of self-suggestion. That's what autogenic training offers. Autogenic training is a relaxation method that uses self-suggestion to guide your body into a state of calm. It's all about focusing inward, using visual imagery and body awareness to reduce stress and create a deep sense of relaxation. It's a way to help your body feel more relaxed by paying attention to things like your breath or heartbeat.

According to the American Psychological Association, autogenic training is a proven technique for stress reduction. By shifting your focus away from the external chaos of life and toward the internal sensations of your body, you can create a peaceful, calming effect that helps you manage stress more effectively.

How to Practice Autogenic Training

Let's walk through a simple way to get started with autogenic training. This technique is perfect for beginners and can be easily incorporated into your daily routine.

1. **Set the Scene:**

    - Find a quiet spot where you can sit or lie down comfortably. This could be your favorite chair, your bed, or even a cozy spot on the floor. Take a few moments to settle in and get comfortable.

2. **Focus on Your Breath:**

    - Start by focusing on your breathing. Notice the gentle rise and fall of your chest or the sensation of air passing through your nostrils. Let your breath be your anchor, grounding you in the present moment.

3. **Visualize Calm:**

   ○ As you breathe, create a calming image in your mind. Picture yourself in a peaceful meadow, surrounded by soft grass and the gentle warmth of the sun. Or imagine the soothing rhythm of ocean waves lapping at the shore. Let this image flow with your breath, deepening your sense of relaxation.

4. **Repeat Calming Phrases:**

   ○ As you breathe and visualize, silently repeat a calming phrase that resonates with you, such as, "I am calm and at peace." This repetition helps reinforce the relaxation response and anchors your mind in serenity.

5. **Make It a Habit:**

   ○ The more you practice, the more effective autogenic training becomes. Try to incorporate it into your daily routine—whether it's a dedicated session each day or a quick moment of calm during a busy afternoon.

Getting Started: Professional Help or DIY?

You can choose to work with a trained professional who can guide you through structured autogenic training sessions tailored to your needs. If you prefer to explore on your own, there are plenty of resources available, like those from the British Autogenic Society, which offer detailed guides and exercises for practicing independently. Autogenic training is like painting calmness across your mind and body, one breath at a time. By practicing this technique, you'll manage stress better and discover a deeper sense of peace within yourself. So why not give it a try? With each session, you're crafting a more serene, balanced inner world, one breath, one thought, and one peaceful moment at a time.

Biofeedback: Listen to Your Body

Ever wish you could tap into your body's natural rhythms and learn to control things like stress, tension, or even your heart rate? That's exactly what biofeedback offers, a technique that helps you listen to your body and take charge of your physiological processes to promote relaxation and reduce stress.

Biofeedback is like having a backstage pass to your own body. It's a mind-body technique that allows you to tune into the signals your body is sending you. By paying attention to signals from your heart rate, blood pressure, muscle tension, skin temperature, and more, you can learn to manage them more effectively, leading to a calmer, more relaxed you.

How Biofeedback Works

Imagine your body as an orchestra, with biofeedback as the conductor guiding each instrument to play in harmony. According to the Cleveland Clinic, biofeedback is a practice that helps you gain mastery over your body's functions. By providing real-time insights into your physiological processes, biofeedback acts as a compass, helping you navigate stress and find your way to relaxation.

In the past, biofeedback required specialized equipment and professional guidance. But thanks to modern technology, it's now more accessible than ever. Home biofeedback devices and apps like emWave2 and Muse have made it easy for beginners to explore this technique right from the comfort of their own homes. These tools monitor your heart rate variability (HRV), a key indicator of stress, and help you use techniques like deep breathing to promote relaxation.

How to Get Started with Biofeedback

Let's dive into how you can use biofeedback to create your own personal calm:

1. **Set Up Your Device:**

    - Start by setting up your home biofeedback device. Make sure it's connected properly and ready to provide real-time feedback. Whether it's a wearable or a handheld device, comfort is key.

2. **Monitor Heart Rate Variability:**

    - Focus on monitoring your heart rate variability (HRV), which shows how your body responds to stress. Watch how your heart rate changes and learn to recognize the patterns.

3. **Practice Deep Breathing:**

    - As you observe your HRV, start practicing deep breathing exercises. The device will give you visual or auditory cues to help guide the pace of your breath. Inhale deeply, hold for a moment, and then exhale slowly, letting the feedback guide you.

4. **Adjust Based on Feedback:**

    - Pay attention to the real-time feedback from your device. If your heart rate is still elevated, try slowing down your breathing or relaxing your muscles even more. The goal is to align your body's responses with a state of calm.

5. **Make It a Habit:**

   - Consistency is key. Incorporate biofeedback into your daily routine, whether it's a few minutes each morning or a longer session before bed. The more you practice, the better you'll become at controlling your physiological responses and achieving relaxation.

Biofeedback isn't just a technique; it's a journey of self-discovery. As you explore the rhythms of your body, you'll become more attuned to its signals and learn how to respond in ways that promote calm and well-being.

Gratitude Journaling

Setting aside a few minutes daily to record three specific things you're grateful for and reflecting on why each item brings joy can enhance the depth of your gratitude. Here, we envision your gratitude journal as a treasure map, unlocking positive experiences:

- **Treasure Entries:** Each gratitude entry is like discovering a treasure on your map. Be specific about the elements that bring you joy, treating them as valuable findings.

- **Revisiting Richness:** Revisiting your entries is akin to retracing your steps on the treasure map. Uncover the richness of positive experiences embedded in each gratitude moment.

- **Mindset Shift Exploration:** See your gratitude journal as a tool for exploring a mindset shift. Every entry contributes to the evolving landscape of positivity and appreciation.

By infusing creativity into your gratitude journaling, you transform it into an engaging and rewarding practice that deepens your connection with the positive aspects of life.

Lifestyle Changes

Introducing small, sustainable lifestyle changes can create an environment where chronic stress is lowered. This might include incorporating daily walks, adjusting sleep patterns, or establishing dedicated tech-free zones. For example, you can use the following steps to elevate your daily walk into a mindful journey, turning it into a sensory adventure:

- **Texture Exploration:** Feel the ground beneath your feet. Notice the textures—whether it's soft grass, cool pavement, or uneven terrain. Engage your sense of touch, connecting with the earth beneath you.

- **Scent Awareness:** Inhale deeply and discern the scents around you. Identify the subtle fragrances of flowers, the earthiness of soil, or the freshness of the air. Let each breath be an opportunity to immerse yourself in the olfactory richness of your surroundings.

- **Color Appreciation:** Observe the colors that paint your path. Notice the vibrant hues of nature, the play of light and shadow, and the palette of the sky. Let the visual spectrum become a source of wonder and appreciation.

- **Slow-Paced Exploration:** Shift into a slower pace, treating your walk as a mini-adventure. Explore the world around you at a leisurely speed, allowing moments of presence to unfold.

Mindful walking creates a heightened sense of being in the present moment, while engaging your senses can help alleviate stress and promote relaxation. Appreciating textures, scents, and colors deepens your connection with the natural world. By infusing mindfulness into your daily walk, you transform it into a rich and rejuvenating experience, allowing you to savor the beauty that surrounds you.

The key to sustaining any lifestyle change is to experiment, discover what resonates with you, and tailor strategies to your unique preferences and needs.

9

Nightly Nurturing: the Role of Sleep in Mental Health

Did you know that lack of proper sleep can amplify the effects of anxiety and depression? It's easy to overlook the crucial role that proper sleep plays in our overall well-being, but it is a powerful tool acting as a natural mood regulator. In this chapter we will explore the ways in which we can prioritize our sleep and provide nightly nurturing for ourselves, to ensure we are taking care of our mental health as well as we do our physical health. So turn off your devices, grab a cup of chamomile tea, and let's explore the magic of sleep.

The Sleep-Mental Health Connection

Sleep and mental health are inherently interconnected. Research has shown that lack of sleep can exacerbate symptoms of anxiety and depression, while good sleep habits can help manage these conditions (Bean and Richey, 2013; Chapman et al., 2013; Short et al., 2013; Xu et al., 2011). The National Sleep Foundation found that those suffering from insomnia are at a significantly higher risk of developing depression than those who sleep well. In fact, their risk is ten times higher!

The importance of getting high-quality sleep simply cannot be overstated when it comes to maintaining good mental health. By prioritizing a healthy sleep routine, many people suffering from anxiety and depression may be able to reduce the severity of their symptoms and improve their overall wellbeing.

Sleep is a vital component of our overall well-being, allowing our brains to rest and recharge after a long day. It improves our ability to manage stress, make decisions, and control our emotions, and serves as a crucial time for the body to support healthy brain function and maintain physical health. This is especially important for children and teens, as sleep plays a key role in supporting their growth and development. Unfortunately, a lack of sleep can have serious consequences, resulting in impulsive behavior, mood swings, and an increased risk of accidents. It's clear that making sleep a priority is essential for both our mental and physical health.

The Impact of Anxiety and Depression on Sleep

When it comes to mental health, it's important to recognize that issues like anxiety and depression can often have a domino effect on other areas of our lives. One such area is our sleep. Unfortunately, anxiety and depression can create a vicious cycle where poor sleep leads to worse anxiety and depression, which in turn leads to even more disrupted sleep.

For example, individuals with generalized anxiety disorder may find themselves unable to quiet their racing thoughts at bedtime, leading to difficulty falling asleep or staying asleep throughout the night. In fact, research from the Anxiety and Depression Association of America tells us that more than half of adults in the United States with this disorder report experiencing sleep problems. This underscores the importance of addressing both mental health and sleep issues simultaneously in order to break the cycle and improve overall well-being.

Depression can be a debilitating mental illness that can manifest itself in various ways. One of the most common symptoms is disrupted sleep patterns. According to the National Institute of Mental Health, individuals with depression often experience insomnia and may find themselves waking up in the early hours of the morning, unable to drift back to sleep. On the other hand, some individuals with depression may be plagued with hypersomnia, excessive sleepiness, and struggle to get out of bed.

Both of these sleep disturbances can affect a person's daily life significantly, leaving them feeling fatigued, irritable, and struggling to function. Depression can take a significant toll on a person's mental and physical health, but with the proper treatment, individuals can learn to sleep better and manage their depression more effectively.

Practical Tips for Improving Sleep Hygiene with Anxiety and Depression

Good sleep hygiene, which means creating habits that support consistent, restful sleep, can make a world of difference in managing anxiety and depression. Here are some practical tips to help you get the rest you need:

1. Stick to a Consistent Sleep Schedule. Your body loves routine, so help it out by going to bed and waking up at the same time every day, even on weekends. This consistency helps regulate your internal clock, making it easier to fall asleep and wake up naturally.

2. Create a Relaxing Pre-Sleep Routine. Ease into bedtime with activities that calm your mind and body. This could be reading a book, taking a warm bath, listening to some chill tunes, or practicing relaxation exercises. These rituals signal to your body that it's time to unwind and prepare for sleep.

3. Craft a Sleep-Friendly Environment. Make your bedroom a sanctuary for sleep. Keep it cool, dark, and quiet. Consider investing in a comfortable mattress and pillows that suit your needs. If noise or light is a problem, think about using earplugs, an eye mask, or a white noise machine to create the perfect sleep setting.

4. Cut Down on Screen Time Before Bed. The blue light from screens can mess with your melatonin production, which is the hormone that helps you sleep. Try to turn off your electronics at least an hour before bed to help your body wind down naturally.

5. Be Mindful of What You Eat and Drink. What you consume in the evening can impact your sleep. Avoid large meals, caffeine, and nicotine close to bedtime, as they can keep you tossing and turning. Opt for a light snack if you're hungry, and stick to water or herbal tea.

6. Stay Active, But Time It Right. Exercise is great for improving sleep quality, but try to get your workout in earlier in the day. Exercising too close to bedtime can rev up your energy levels, making it harder to fall asleep.

7. Manage Stress with Relaxation Techniques. Incorporate relaxation exercises like deep breathing, meditation, or gentle yoga into your nighttime routine. These practices can calm your mind, reduce anxiety, and set the stage for a restful night.

8. Soak Up Some Sunlight. Exposure to natural light, especially in the morning, helps regulate your body's internal clock and can improve your sleep quality. Try to spend some time outside each day, or at least near a window.

9. Keep Naps Short and Sweet. While a quick nap can be refreshing, avoid taking long or late-afternoon naps. These can throw off your sleep schedule and make it harder to fall asleep at night.

10. Don't Hesitate to Seek Professional Help. If you're still struggling with sleep, it might be time to talk to a healthcare professional. They can help identify any underlying issues and provide personalized recommendations or treatments.

Improving your sleep hygiene is an investment in your overall well-being. By integrating these practical tips into your routine, you can create an environment and lifestyle that supports better sleep. Remember, the key to better sleep is consistency and making small, manageable changes. Here's to better sleep and brighter days ahead!

Busting Common Sleep Myths: Let's Set the Record Straight

When it comes to sleep, there are a lot of myths floating around that can lead to misunderstandings of what's good for our health. Let's tackle some of the big ones so you can sleep better and feel better!

Myth 1: "I Can Just Catch Up on Sleep over the Weekend"

We've all been there, pulling late nights during the week and telling ourselves we'll catch up on sleep over the weekend. But here's the hard truth: you can't really "catch up" on lost sleep. Researchers at Harvard Medical School have shown that missing out on sleep can leave lasting effects on your mood and cognitive abilities, and you can't just erase those effects by sleeping in on Saturday. It's much better to aim for consistent, good-quality sleep every night rather than trying to make up for it later.

Myth 2: "Older Adults Need Less Sleep"

There's a common belief that as we get older, we don't need as much sleep. But according to the National Sleep Foundation, adults of all ages still need about seven to nine hours of sleep each night to stay healthy. Sure, your sleep patterns might change as you age—for instance, you might go to bed earlier or wake up earlier—but the need for quality sleep doesn't decrease. So, whether you're twenty-five or seventy-five, getting those seven to nine hours is still key to feeling your best.

Myth 3: "Snoring Is Just Annoying, Not Harmful"

Snoring might seem like a harmless, if annoying, part of life, but it can actually be a red flag for something more serious: sleep apnea. Sleep apnea is a sleep disorder where breathing repeatedly stops and starts during the night, which can lead to a whole host of health problems, including issues with your heart and lungs. If you or someone you know is a frequent, loud snorer, it might be time to see a doctor. Don't just brush it off because getting it checked out could be a game-changer for your health.

Understanding the truth about sleep is the first step toward improving your health and well-being. By debunking these myths, you can focus on what really matters—getting consistent, high-quality sleep. So let's stop believing the hype and start giving our sleep the attention it deserves. After all, a good night's sleep is one of the best gifts you can give yourself!

Conclusion

The journey through anxiety and depression is complex, but it's also deeply personal—and healing looks different for everyone. Over these chapters, we've explored the biological roots of mental health; the various disorders associated with anxiety and depression; the importance of addressing stress before it becomes overwhelming; available medications and their pros and cons; and the power of nutrition, mindfulness, movement, and sleep. Together these elements form a holistic approach, reminding us that no single solution fits all but that every small step matters.

The path forward requires patience, self-compassion, and a willingness to try, fail, and try again. Healing is not about perfection but about progress—finding what works for you and leaning into practices that nurture your mind, body, and spirit. Whether you're taking your first step or have been on this journey for some time, know that you are not alone. There is light within you, waiting to be cultivated. With time, support, and self-care, a life of balance and peace is not just possible—it's within reach. Keep going, and trust the process.

SPREADING HOPE, ONE REVIEW AT A TIME

Now that you've explored *Understanding Anxiety and Depression* and gained tools to navigate mental health challenges, it's time to share your insights and help others discover the same guidance.

By leaving your honest opinion of this book on Amazon, you'll show others who are struggling with anxiety and depression where they can find support and hope.

Your review could be the encouragement someone needs to take a step toward healing and understanding.

To leave a review, click here!

Thank you for helping us continue this important mission. Together, we can ensure that hope and knowledge reach those who need it most.

Your voice matters, and your kindness in sharing it is deeply appreciated.

To Health & Healing,
Dr. A

References

Amsterdam, J. D., Shults, J., Soeller, I., Rockwell, K., Mao, J. J., & Viniegra-Rodriguez, G. (2009). Chamomile (Matricaria recutita) may have modest benefits for generalized anxiety disorder: A randomized controlled trial. *Phytomedicine, 16*(5), 344-348.

Anxiety and Depression Association of America (ADAA). (n.d.). Anxiety and sleep. Retrieved from

Bandelow, B., Reitt, M., Röver, C., Michaelis, S., Görlich, Y., & Wedekind, D. (2015). Efficacy of treatments for anxiety disorders: A meta-analysis. *International Clinical Psychopharmacology, 30*(4), 183–192.

Bayes, J., Schloss, J., & Sibbritt, D. (2022). The effect of a Mediterranean diet on the symptoms of depression in young males (the "AMMEND" study): A Randomized Control Trial. *The American Journal of Clinical Nutrition.*

Bean, J. L., & Richey, J. A. (2013). Naturalistic partial sleep deprivation leads to greater next-day anxiety: The moderating role of baseline anxiety and depression. *Journal of Sleep Research, 22*(4), 476-485.

Blanck, P., Perleth, S., Heidenreich, T., Kröger, P., Ditzen, B., Bents, H., & Mander, J. (2018). Effects of mindfulness exercises as stand-alone intervention on symptoms of anxiety and depression: Systematic review and meta-analysis. *Behaviour Research and Therapy, 102*, 25-35.

Bremner, J. D. (2006). Traumatic stress: effects on the brain. *Dialogues in clinical neuroscience*, *8*(4), 445-461.

Celano, C. M., Daunis, D. J., Lokko, H. N., Campbell, K. A., & Huffman, J. C. (2016). Anxiety disorders and cardiovascular disease. *Current psychiatry reports, 18*, 1-11.

Chapman, D. P., Wheaton, A. G., Anda, R. F., Croft, J. B., Edwards, V. J., Liu, Y., & Perry, G. S. (2013). Frequent insufficient sleep and anxiety and depressive disorders among U.S. community dwellers in 20 states, 2010. *Sleep Medicine, 14*(8), 778-784.

Chu, B., Marwaha, K., Sanvictores, T., & Ayers, D. (2019). Physiology, stress reaction.

Colman, I., Ploubidis, G. B., Wadsworth, M. E., Jones, P. B., & Croudace, T. J. (2007). A longitudinal typology of symptoms of depression and anxiety over the life course. *Biological psychiatry, 62*(11), 1265-1271.

Côté, S. M., Boivin, M., Liu, X., Nagin, D. S., Zoccolillo, M., & Tremblay, R. E. (2009). Depression and anxiety symptoms: onset, developmental course and risk factors during early childhood. *Journal of Child Psychology and Psychiatry, 50*(10), 1201-1208.

Craske, M. G., & Barlow, D. H. (2006). *Mastery of your anxiety and worry.* Oxford University Press.

Diego, M. A., Jones, N. A., Field, T., Hernandez-Reif, M., Schanberg, S., Kuhn, C., & McAdam, V. (1998). Aromatherapy positively affects mood, EEG patterns of alertness and math computations. *International Journal of Neuroscience, 96*(3-4), 217-224.

Dimidjian, S., Hollon, S. D., Dobson, K. S., Schmaling, K. B., Kohlenberg, R. J., Addis, M. E., Gallop, R., McGlinchey, J. B., Markley, D. K., Gollan, J. K., Atkins, D. C., Dunner, D. L., & Jacobson, N. S. (2006). Randomized trial of behavioral activation, cognitive therapy, and antidepressant medication in the acute treatment of adults with major depression. *Journal of Consulting and Clinical Psychology, 74*(4), 658-670.

Everly, Jr, G. S., Lating, J. M., Everly, G. S., & Lating, J. M. (2019). The anatomy and physiology of the human stress response. *A clinical guide to the treatment of the human stress response*, 19-56.

Facts & Statistics | Anxiety and Depression Association of America, ADAA. (n.d.).

Forsyth, J. P., & Eifert, G. H. (2016). *The mindfulness and acceptance workbook for anxiety: A guide to breaking free from anxiety, phobias, and worry using acceptance and commitment therapy.* New Harbinger Publications.

Golden, R. N., Gaynes, B. N., Ekstrom, R. D., Hamer, R. M., Jacobsen, F. M., Suppes, T., Wisner, K. L., & Nemeroff, C. B. (2005). The efficacy of light therapy in the treatment of mood disorders: a review and meta-analysis of the evidence. *The American Journal of Psychiatry, 162*(4), 656-662.

Goyal, M., Singh, S., Sibinga, E. M. S., Gould, N. F., Rowland-Seymour, A., Sharma, R., ... &

Haythornthwaite, J. A. (2014). Meditation programs for psychological stress and well-being: A systematic review and meta-analysis. *JAMA Internal Medicine, 174*(3), 357-368.

Hofmann, S. G., Wu, J. Q., & Boettcher, H. (2014). Effect of cognitive-behavioral therapy for anxiety disorders on quality of life: a meta-analysis. *Journal of consulting and clinical psychology, 82*(3), 375.

Hongratanaworakit, T. (2004). Effects of inhalation of essential oils on EEG activity and sensory evaluation—investigating lavender and ylang-ylang. *Phytotherapy Research, 18*(12), 977-981.

Johnson, E. O., Kamilaris, T. C., Chrousos, G. P., & Gold, P. W. (1992). Mechanisms of stress: a dynamic overview of hormonal and behavioral homeostasis. *Neuroscience & Biobehavioral Reviews, 16*(2), 115-130.

Kaczkurkin, A. N., & Foa, E. B. (2015). Cognitive-behavioral therapy for anxiety disorders: an update on the empirical evidence. *Dialogues in clinical neuroscience, 17*(3), 337-346.

Kasper, S., Gastpar, M., Müller, W. E., Volz, H. P., Möller, H. J., & Dienel, A. (2010). Efficacy of Silexan in anxiety-related restlessness and disturbed sleep—a randomized, placebo-controlled trial. *European Neuropsychopharmacology, 20*(10), 738-746.

Kuyken, W., Hayes, R., Barrett, B., Byng, R., Dalgleish, T., Kessler, D., ... & Croudace, T. J. (2015). Mindfulness-based cognitive therapy to prevent relapse in recurrent depression. *The Lancet, 386*(9988), 63-73.

Lespérance, F., Frasure-Smith, N., St-André, E., Turecki, G., Lespérance, P., & Wisniewski, S. (2011). The efficacy of omega-3 supplementation for major depression: A randomized controlled trial. *The Journal of Clinical Psychiatry, 72*(8), 1054-1062.

Luppino, F. S., de Wit, L. M., Bouvy, P. F., Stijnen, T., Cuijpers, P., Penninx, B. W., & Zitman, F. G. (2010). Overweight, obesity, and depression: a systematic review and meta-analysis of longitudinal studies. *Archives of general psychiatry, 67*(3), 220-229.

Ma, X., Yue, Z. Q., Gong, Z. Q., Zhang, H., Duan, N. Y., Shi, Y. T., ... & Li, Y. F. (2017). The effect of diaphragmatic breathing on attention, negative affect and stress in healthy adults. *Frontiers in psychology, 8*, 234806.

Major Depression. (n.d.). National Institute of Mental Health (NIMH). https://www.nimh.nih.gov/health/statistics/major-depression

Martens, E. J., de Jonge, P., Na, B., Cohen, B. E., Lett, H., & Whooley, M. A. (2010). Scared to death? Generalized anxiety disorder and cardiovascular events in patients with stable coronary heart disease: *The Heart and Soul Study. Archives of general psychiatry, 67*(7), 750-758.

McLaughlin, K. A. (2011). The public health impact of major depression: a call for interdisciplinary prevention efforts. *Prevention Science, 12,* 361-371.

Murphy, P. K., & Wagner, C. (2008). Vitamin D and mood disorders among women: an integrative review. *Journal of Midwifery & Women's Health, 53*(5), 440-446.

National Institute of Mental Health (NIMH). (n.d.). Depression basics. Retrieved from

Newman, M. G. (2000). Recommendations for a cost-offset model of psychotherapy allocation using generalized anxiety disorder as an example. *Journal of consulting and clinical psychology, 68*(4), 549.

Otte, C. (2011). Cognitive behavioral therapy in anxiety disorders: Current state of the evidence. *Dialogues in Clinical Neuroscience, 13*(4), 413-421.

Peirce, J. M., & Alviña, K. (2019). The role of inflammation and the gut microbiome in depression and anxiety. *Journal of Neuroscience Research, 97*(10), 1223-1241.

Professional, C. C. M. (n.d.). *Serotonin*. Cleveland Clinic.

Purse, M. (2023, November 8). *Techniques to tame the Fight-or-Flight response*. Verywell Mind. .

Robinson, O. J., Vytal, K., Cornwell, B. R., & Grillon, C. (2013). The impact of anxiety upon cognition: perspectives from human threat of shock studies. *Frontiers in human neuroscience, 7*, 203.

Saeedi, M., & Rashidy-Pour, A. (2021). Association between chronic stress and Alzheimer's disease: Therapeutic effects of Saffron. *Biomedicine & Pharmacotherapy, 133*, 110995.

Savas, L. S., White, D. L., Wieman, M., Daci, K., Fitzgerald, S., Laday Smith, S., ... & EL-SERAG, H. B. (2009). Irritable bowel syndrome and dyspepsia among women veterans: prevalence and association with psychological distress. *Alimentary pharmacology & therapeutics, 29*(1), 115-125.

Shallua, L. D. (2024). *Priorities of life: Putting first things first*. [Paperback].

Sherman, S. M., & Guillery, R. W. (2006). *Exploring the thalamus and its role in cortical function* (2nd ed.). Cambridge, MA: MIT Press.

Short, M. A., Gradisar, M., Lack, L. C., Wright, H. R., & Dohnt, H. (2013). Sleep deprivation leads to mood deficits in healthy adolescents. *Sleep Medicine*, 14(9), 849-856.

Silva, J.E., Castilhas, J.H., Sousa, S.C., Guimarães, A.S., Gama, J.P., Sousa, L.C., Moreira, L.C., Ribeiro, M.M., Menelli, H.P., Penha, T.P., Reis, M.A., & Silveira, M. (2023). THE ROLE OF VITAMIN D IN THE DEVELOPMENT/WORSEAGE OF MOOD DISORDERS, WITH A FOCUS ON BIPOLAR AFFECTIVE DISORDER AND DEPRESSION. *International Journal of Health Science*.

Snel, M., Gastaldelli, A., Ouwens, D., Hesselink, M., Schaart, G., Buzzigoli, E., ... & Jazet, I. (2012). Effects of adding exercise to a 16-week very low-calorie diet in obese, insulin-dependent type 2 diabetes mellitus patients. *The Journal of Clinical Endocrinology and Metabolism*, 97(7), 2512-2520.

Srivastava, J. K., Shankar, E., & Gupta, S. (2010). Chamomile: A herbal medicine of the past with a bright future (Review). *Molecular Medicine Reports*, 3(6), 895-901.

Stangor, C. (2014, October 17). *4.2 Our brains control our thoughts, feelings, and behaviour*. Pressbooks.

Toussaint, L., Nguyen, Q. A., Roettger, C., Dixon, K., Offenbächer, M., Kohls, N., Hirsch, J., & Sirois, F. (2021). Effectiveness of Progressive Muscle Relaxation, Deep Breathing, and Guided Imagery in Promoting Psychological and Physiological States of Relaxation. Evidence-based complementary and alternative medicine : eCAM, 2021, 5924040.

Trivedi, M. H. (2004). The link between depression and physical symptoms. *Primary care companion to the Journal of clinical psychiatry*, 6(suppl 1), 12.

Tylee, A., & Gandhi, P. (2005). The importance of somatic symptoms in depression in primary care. *Primary care companion to the Journal of clinical psychiatry*, 7(4), 167.

Wagner, J. (1985). *The Search for Signs of Intelligent Life in the Universe.* [Broadway Play]

Wittchen, H. U. (2002). Generalized anxiety disorder: prevalence, burden, and cost to society. *Depression and anxiety, 16*(4), 162-171.

Xu, L., Jiang, C. Q., & Lam, T. H. (2011). The role of depression and anxiety in the relationship between poor sleep quality and subjective cognitive decline in Chinese elderly. *Sleep Medicine,* 12(9), 815-820.

Yang, C. C., Barrós-Loscertales, A., Li, M., Pinazo, D., Borchardt, V., Ávila, C., & Walter, M. (2019). Alterations in brain structure and amplitude of low-frequency after 8 weeks of mindfulness meditation training in meditation-naïve subjects. *Scientific Reports, 9*(1), 10977.

Yaribeygi, H., Panahi, Y., Sahraei, H., Johnston, T. P., & Sahebkar, A. (2017). The impact of stress on body function: A review. *EXCLI journal, 16,* 1057.

www.ingramcontent.com/pod-product-compliance
Lightning Source LLC
Chambersburg PA
CBHW020543030426
42337CB00013B/961